THE SCIENCE OF WEIGHT LOSS MANAGEMENT

Table of Contents:

Introduction--- 5

Chapter 1: Understanding Weight Loss -------------------------------------6 to 8

    1.1 The Science Behind Weight Loss

    1.2 Metabolism and Energy Balance

    1.3 Setting Realistic Goals

Chapter 2: Nutrition Essentials---9 to 11

    2.1 Macronutrients: Carbs, Proteins, and Fats

    2.2 Micronutrients: Vitamins and Minerals
    2.3 Hydration and Its Role in Weight Management

Chapter 3: Mindful Eating--12 to 16

    3.1 The Psychology of Eating

    3.2 Mindful Eating Techniques
    3.3 Overcoming Emotional Eating

Chapter 4: Exercise and Movement---17 to24

    4.1 Benefits of Physical Activity

    4.2 Finding Your Exercise Routine
    4.3 Incorporating Movement Into Daily Life

Chapter 5: Building Healthy Habits--25 to 44

    5.1 The Power of Habits

    5.2 Strategies for Building Healthy Habits

    5.3 Overcoming Obstacles and Staying Consistent

Chapter 6: Sleep and Stress Management-------------------------------------45 to 49

    6.1 Importance of Sleep for Weight Loss

    6.2 Strategies for Improving Sleep Quality
    6.3 Managing Stress for Weight Management

Chapter 7: Tracking Progress---50 to 52

    7.1 Tracking Food Intake

    7.2 Monitoring Physical Activity
    7.3 Celebrating Non-Scale Victories

Chapter 8: Overcoming Plateaus and Setbacks----------------------------------53 to 62

    8.1 Understanding Weight Loss Plateaus

    8.2 Strategies for Breaking Through Plateaus

    8.3 Dealing with Setbacks

Chapter 9: Building a Support System --63 to 66

    9.1 Importance of Social Support

    9.2 Finding Accountability Partners

    9.3 Seeking Professional Support

Chapter 10: Long-Term Maintenance---67 to 69

    10.1 Transitioning to Maintenance--------------------------------

    10.2 Strategies for Preventing Weight Regain--------------------

    10.3 Making Health a Lifestyle------------------------------------

Chapter 11: Setting Realistic Goals--70 to 81

    1. Define Specific and Clear Goals ---

    2. Evaluate Your Resources and Limitations----------------------------

    3. Break Goals Down into Smaller Steps--------------------------------

    4. Create a Timeline that is Realistic-------------------------------------

    5. Maintain your flexibility and adaptability--------------------------

    6. Plan and Prepare Meals--

    7. Pay attention to your own body-------------------------------------

Chapter 12: Physical activity and exercise--82 to 86

    Importance of Physical Activity---------------------------------------

    1. Improves Cardiovascular Health--

    2. Weight Management---

    3. Improved mental health--

    4. Increased Muscle and Bone Strength------------------------------------

    5. Better Sleep Quality--

Chapter 13: Tips for Implementing Physical Activity and Exercise---------87 to 91

1. Find Activities That You Enjoy---

2. Begin slowly and progress gradually--

3. Set Realistic Goals--

4. Add Variety--

5. Make It Social---

6. Prioritize Consistency---

7. Listen to Your Body--

Chapter 14: Mindset and Behavior Changes------------------------------------92 to 93

Understanding Mindsets: ---

1. The Fixed Mindset ---

2. The Growth Mindset ---

3. The effect of mindset on behavior change------------------------------------

Chapter 15: Promoting a Growth Mindset--94

1. Be open to challenges---

2. See Effort as the Path to Mastery---

3. Get Feedback--

4. Recognize and celebrate growth and progress-------------------------------

Chapter 16: Behavior Change: The Path to Transformation---------------------95 to 98

1. Set Clear and Achievable Goals---

2. Identify Triggers and Barriers--

3. Create a Supportive Environment--

4. Develop Self-Compassion---

5. Be Consistent and Persistent ---

Chapter 17: Combining Mindset and Behavior Change----------------------------99 to 102

1. Mindset ---

2. Behavioral Change--

Chapter 18: Conclusion--103 to 104

Introduction:

Starting your quest to achieve your ideal weight is a critical step toward enhancing your overall health and well-being. In a world filled with fad diets, conflicting advice, and quick-fix solutions, it's vital to approach weight loss in a balanced and informed manner.

This journey is about more than just hitting a number on a scale; it is about creating a sustainable lifestyle that supports your long-term health goals.

Knowing that each person's ideal weight is unique and governed by features such as body composition, muscle mass, and genetic predisposition underscores the importance of personalized

Weight-management techniques. Rather than chasing ethereal ideals or cultural standards, the focus should be on cultivating a balanced relationship with food, physical activity, and self-care.

Beginning your journey to obtain your target weight is an important step towards improving your overall health and well-being. In a world full of fad diets, contradicting advice, and quick fixes, it's critical to approach weight loss in a balanced and informed way.

This journey is about more than just achieving a number on a scale; it is about developing a sustainable lifestyle that supports your long-term health objectives.

The fact that each person's optimal weight is unique and determined by variables such as body composition, muscle mass, and genetic predisposition highlights the need of tailored

Weight-management strategies. Rather than pursuing ethereal ideals or cultural standards, the goal should be to cultivate a healthy relationship with diet, physical activity, and self-care.

Chapter 1: Understanding Your Ideal Weight:

Before commencing on any weight loss quest, you must first determine your optimum weight. This is more than just aiming at a specific number on the scale. Body composition, muscular mass, and overall health all play an important impact.

Consulting with a healthcare expert or qualified dietitian can assist you in determining a realistic and healthy weight target based on your specific circumstances.

Maintaining the right weight is critical for general health and well-being. However, determining what constitutes an optimal weight can be difficult and individualized.

Rather than relying exclusively on social standards or body mass index (BMI), it is critical to examine a variety of factors when establishing your optimal weight.

To begin, acknowledge that everyone's optimal weight varies depending on their height, body composition, muscle mass, bone density, and genetic predisposition.

Rather than aiming for a specific number on the scale, aim for a weight that allows you to feel energetic, strong, and at ease in your body.

In addition, work for a balanced lifestyle that includes regular physical activity, nutritious eating habits, stress management, and appropriate sleep. These lifestyle habits have a substantial impact on weight management and overall well-being.

Rather of chasing unachievable goals, focus on long-term health-promoting practices. Consult with a healthcare professional, such as a nutritionist or a doctor, to create individualized methods for achieving and maintaining your desired weight.

Remember, the journey to your ideal weight is not solely about numbers but about fostering a positive relationship with your body and prioritizing your health and happiness.

By understanding and embracing your unique needs and striving for balance, you can achieve and maintain your ideal weight in a healthy and sustainable manner.

1.1 The Science Behind Weight Loss

The fundamental notion of energy balance serves as the foundation for weight loss research. At its essence, weight loss happens when the number of calories taken is fewer than the number of calories burned by the body.

This notion, known as "calories in, calories out," serves as the foundation for most weight management plans. The human body requires energy to execute basic processes such as breathing, blood circulation, and body temperature regulation.

This baseline energy expenditure is known as the basal metabolic rate (BMR), and it accounts for the vast majority of calories burned each day. In addition to the BMR, energy is expended through physical activity and the thermic effect of food, which is the energy necessary to digest, absorb, and metabolise

To lose weight, people must establish a calorie deficit by either reducing their calorie intake, increasing their physical activity, or a combination of both. This deficit drives the body to draw on its stored energy reserves, primarily fat, resulting in weight reduction over time.

However, the science of weight loss goes beyond mere calorie counting. Macronutrient content, meal timing, hormone modulation, and individual metabolic variances are all important factors in determining weight loss effectiveness.

Understanding these components and how they interact with one another is critical for creating effective and long-term weight loss solutions.

1.2 Metabolism and Energy Balance

Metabolism and energy balance are important principles for understanding weight management and overall health. Metabolism refers to the complicated metabolic processes that take place within the body to transform food into energy. This energy is used to power vital operations like respiration, circulation, and cellular repair.

The basal metabolic rate (BMR) is the least amount of energy required to maintain these essential body functions while at rest. Age, gender, body composition, and heredity all have an impact on an individual's basal metabolic rate. Physical activity and food's thermal effect also contribute to overall energy expenditure.

To achieve and maintain a healthy weight, you must strike a balance between energy intake (calories consumed) and energy expenditure (calories burned). When energy intake exceeds expenditure, the body stores extra calories as fat, resulting in weight gain.

When energy expenditure exceeds intake, the body must use stored fat as fuel, which causes weight loss. Diet composition, physical activity level, sleep quality, and stress levels are all factors that might have an impact on metabolism and energy balance.

Individuals can improve their metabolism and maintain a healthy weight over time by adopting healthy lifestyle behaviors such as eating a well-balanced diet, exercising regularly, getting enough sleep, and managing stress efficiently. Understanding the interplay of metabolism and energy balance is key for optimal weight management.

1.3 Setting Realistic Goals

Setting realistic objectives is an essential part of succeeding in any pursuit, including weight reduction and fitness. Realistic objectives are those that are attainable and within reach, taking into account one's personal circumstances, abilities, and resources.

When establishing weight loss objectives, it is critical to consider current weight, ideal weight, timescale, and lifestyle choices. Setting a realistic target weight that is both healthy and attainable is crucial. This may entail visiting a healthcare practitioner to identify a healthy weight range based on criteria such as height, body composition, and general health.

It is also crucial to set a realistic deadline for achieving your objectives. While quick weight loss may appear tempting, it is frequently unsustainable and might have serious health repercussions. Instead, aiming for moderate, consistent progress—such as dropping 1-2 pounds per week—is more attainable and sustainable in the long run.

Furthermore, adopting behavior-based objectives based on healthy habits rather than just the number on the scale might boost success. Behavior-based goals include exercising for a set amount of time per day, eating a balanced diet rich in fruits and vegetables, and practicing mindful eating behaviors.

Finally, reassessing and revising goals on a frequent basis in response to progress and feedback is critical for staying on track and motivated. Setting realistic goals that are suited to your specific circumstances and focusing on long-term behavior change can improve your chances of attaining long-term success in your weight reduction journey.

Chapter 2: Nutrition Essentials

Nutritional basics are the foundation of a balanced diet and are critical to general well-being. Understanding the fundamentals of nutrition is critical for making sound dietary choices that promote good health and vigor.

Macronutrients are the fundamental components of food that supply energy and nutrition. They consist of carbs, proteins, and lipids. Carbohydrates are the body's major source of energy and can be found in foods such as grains, fruits, and vegetables.

Meat, poultry, fish, lentils, and dairy products are all good sources of protein, which is required for tissue growth and repair. Nuts, seeds, avocados, and oils include fats, which are required for hormone production, cell membrane function, and nutrient absorption.

Micronutrients are vitamins and minerals that are required for many physiological functions in the body. They consist of vitamins A, C, D, E, and K, as well as minerals like calcium, iron, magnesium, and zinc. Micronutrients are essential for metabolism, immunological function, bone health, and many other processes.

Hydration is another important part of nutrition. Water is necessary for appropriate hydration, regulating body temperature, carrying nutrients, and removing waste. Maintaining proper hydration is critical for general health and well-being.

A balanced diet rich in macronutrients, micronutrients, and hydration is critical for maintaining good health, energy levels, and performance in daily living. By prioritizing dietary fundamentals and making thoughtful food choices, individuals can improve their overall quality of life and lower the risk of chronic

2.1 Macronutrients: Carbs, Proteins, and Fats

Macronutrients are the key nutrients that provide the body with energy and are required for survival and numerous physiological activities. Carbohydrates, proteins, and fats are the three primary macronutrients, with each playing a distinct function in general health and well-being.

Carbohydrates are the body's principal source of energy, giving fuel to both the brain and the muscles. Grains, fruits, vegetables, and legumes are all sources of these nutrients. Carbohydrates can be divided into two types:

simple carbohydrates (sugars) and complex carbs (starches and fiber). While simple carbs provide rapid energy, complex carbohydrates provide long-term energy and are necessary for maintaining stable blood sugar levels and encouraging digestive health.

Proteins are required for the development and repair of various tissues, including muscles, organs, and hormones. They are made up of amino acids, which are commonly referred to as protein's "building blocks".

Protein can be obtained from meat, poultry, fish, eggs, dairy products, legumes, nuts, and seeds. An appropriate protein intake is required to sustain muscular growth, immunological function, and overall health.

Fats provide concentrated energy and are required for a variety of body processes such as hormone generation, cell membrane construction, and nutrient absorption. Avocados, almonds, seeds, olive oil, fatty seafood, and coconut oil are examples of healthy fat sources. While fats are frequently derided, integrating healthy fats into the diet is critical for heart health, brain function, and overall well-being.

Consumption of carbs, proteins, and fats must be balanced in order to maintain optimal health and support energy levels, metabolism, and general vitality. Prioritizing whole, nutrient-dense foods while limiting consumption of processed and refined macronutrients can assist improve long-term health and well-being.

2.2 Micronutrients: Vitamins and Minerals

Micronutrients are vital nutrients that the body needs in little amounts to sustain numerous physiological activities and preserve overall health. Vitamins and minerals are the two main types of micronutrients, and they play an important part in a variety of biological processes.

Vitamins are organic chemicals that are required for metabolism, growth, development, and general well-being. Water-soluble vitamins, such as the B vitamins and vitamin C, dissolve in water and are not kept in the body,

whereas fat-soluble vitamins, such as vitamins A, D, E, and K, dissolve in fat and are stored in the liver and fatty tissues. Vitamins work as coenzymes or cofactors in enzymatic reactions, helping to regulate metabolism, support immunological function, and maintain healthy skin, vision, and bones.

Minerals are inorganic elements that are required for many physiological processes, such as bone formation, fluid equilibrium, neuron function, and muscle contraction. They are divided into two types:

macrominerals (calcium, magnesium, phosphorus, sodium, potassium, chloride, and sulfur) and trace minerals (iron, zinc, copper, selenium, iodine, manganese, and chromium), which are required in smaller quantities. Minerals are essential for maintaining electrolyte balance, supporting immunological function, and boosting overall health and wellness.

A diversified and balanced diet rich in vitamins and minerals is critical for maintaining appropriate micronutrient consumption while also promoting optimal health and vigor.
Including a mix of fruits, vegetables, whole grains, lean meats, and healthy fats in your diet will help provide your body with the vitamins and minerals it requires to function properly.

2.3 Hydration and Its Role in Weight Management

Hydration is critical for both weight management and overall health. Water is required for several physiological activities in the body, such as nutrient transport, temperature regulation, waste elimination, and electrolyte balance.

Proper hydration is critical for maintaining metabolism and optimizing the body's capacity to burn calories effectively. Drinking plenty of water can also help with weight loss by increasing feelings of fullness and lowering calorie consumption.

According to studies, drinking water before meals can help lower overall calorie intake, resulting in weight loss over time. Staying hydrated might also help you avoid overeating and snacking because thirst is sometimes misinterpreted for hunger.

Furthermore, enough hydration is critical for exercise performance and recovery. Dehydration can decrease physical performance by reducing endurance, strength, and coordination during exercise sessions.

Individuals who stay properly hydrated can maintain ideal energy levels and performance throughout exercise, resulting in more efficient calorie burning and better weight control outcomes. Consuming hydrating foods such as fruits and vegetables, as well as drinking water throughout the day, is critical for maintaining optimal hydration.

 Monitoring urine color and frequency can also assist determine hydration status, with pale yellow urine indicating sufficient hydration. Individuals can help their weight control and overall well-being by prioritizing hydration as part of a healthy lifestyle.

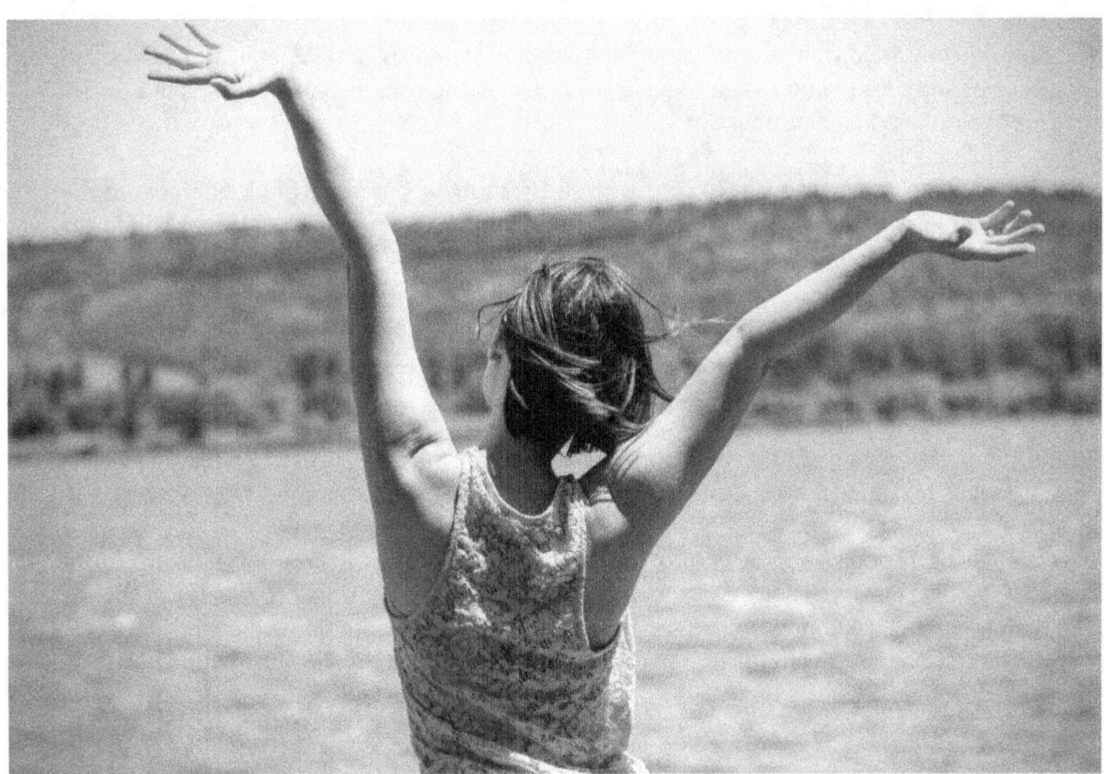

Chapter 3: Mindful Eating

Mindful eating is a discipline that encourages people to focus on the sensory experience of eating without judgment or distraction. It entails being totally present throughout meals, focusing on the flavor, texture, aroma, and even the sound of the food being ingested.

This strategy focuses on internal hunger and satiety cues rather than external indicators like portion size or calorie count. When practicing mindful eating, people take the time to relish each bite, chewing slowly and completely and paying attention to the sensations that develop in their bodies.

This increased awareness can result in a stronger appreciation for food as well as a better knowledge of one's connection with eating. Individuals who practice mindfulness during meals may become more sensitive to their bodies' cues of hunger and fullness, which can help prevent overeating and establish a healthy relationship with food.

In addition to supporting better eating habits, mindful eating has been linked to a variety of additional advantages, including less stress, improved digestion, and enhanced meal satisfaction. Individuals who bring mindfulness to the dinner table can build a stronger feeling of connection with their food and themselves, resulting in a more balanced and rewarding relationship with eating.

3.1 The Psychology of Eating

The psychology of eating delves into the complex interplay between our minds and our relationship with food. It encompasses a wide range of psychological factors that influence our eating habits, attitudes, and behaviors towards food.

This field of study explores how emotions, beliefs, past experiences, and societal influences shape our food choices and consumption patterns. One key aspect of the psychology of eating is understanding the role of emotions in eating behavior.

Many people turn to food as a way to cope with stress, sadness, boredom, or other emotions. Emotional eating can lead to overeating or unhealthy eating habits, as individuals seek comfort or distraction through food.

Another important aspect is the impact of social and cultural influences on eating behavior. Cultural norms, family traditions, peer pressure, and media messages all play a significant role in shaping our food preferences and dietary habits.

Furthermore, the psychology of eating examines individual differences in eating behavior, such as appetite regulation, food cravings, and food preferences. These factors can be influenced by biological, psychological, and environmental factors.

By understanding the psychological factors that drive our eating behavior, individuals can gain insight into their relationship with food and make more informed choices about their diet and lifestyle. This knowledge can also inform interventions and strategies aimed at promoting healthier eating habits and preventing eating disorders.

3.2 Mindful Eating Techniques

Mindful eating techniques involve a variety of practices aimed at fostering a more conscious and intentional approach to eating. These techniques encourage individuals to slow down, tune into their body's hunger and satiety signals, and fully appreciate the sensory experience of eating. Here are some key mindful eating techniques:

1) Mindful Awareness:

Begin by bringing awareness to the present moment before eating. Take a few deep breaths to center yourself and focus your attention on the meal ahead.

Mindful awareness is the deliberate act of paying attention to the present moment without judgment. It entails paying complete attention to our thoughts, feelings, physiological sensations, and the environment around us. People who practice mindful awareness can improve their clarity, focus, and emotional management.

In daily life, attentive awareness can be applied to a variety of activities, including eating, walking, and conversing. By remaining present and attentive in these situations, we can improve our entire experience while reducing tension or anxiety caused by previous regrets or future concerns.

Mindful awareness is an essential component of mindfulness meditation, but it can also be developed through easy daily practices like mindful breathing or body scans. Over time, this practice can result in increased self-awareness, resilience, and a stronger connection to ourselves and the world around us.

2. Slow Down:

Eat slowly and mindfully, taking the time to chew each bite thoroughly and savor the flavors, textures, and aromas of the food. Slowing down while eating food involves consciously taking your time to chew, savor, and fully experience each bite.

It's about being present and attentive to the act of eating rather than rushing through meals mindlessly. By slowing down, you give your body the chance to register feelings of fullness more accurately, which can prevent overeating and promote better digestion.

Slowing down also allows you to appreciate the flavors, textures, and aromas of your food more deeply, enhancing the overall enjoyment of the meal. Additionally, it gives you the opportunity to tune into your body's hunger and satiety cues, helping you develop a healthier relationship with food.

Practicing mindful eating techniques like taking smaller bites, chewing slowly, and putting your fork down between bites can help you slow down and savor your meals. By making a conscious effort to eat more slowly, you may find that you feel more satisfied with less food and experience greater overall satisfaction with your eating experience.

3. Pay Attention:

Tune into your body's hunger and fullness cues throughout the meal. Notice sensations of hunger and satisfaction, and stop eating when you feel comfortably full.

Paying attention while eating food involves being fully present and engaged with the experience of eating. It means focusing your attention on the sensations, flavors, and textures of the food, as well as being aware of your body's hunger and fullness signals.

When you pay attention while eating, you're less likely to eat mindlessly or out of habit. Instead, you're able to make more conscious choices about what and how much you eat. This can lead to better portion control, improved digestion, and a greater appreciation for the food you're consuming.

To practice paying attention while eating, try to minimize distractions such as watching TV or scrolling through your phone. Instead, sit down at a table, take a few deep breaths to center yourself, and focus solely on the act of eating.

Notice the colors, smells, and tastes of your food, and pay attention to how each bite makes you feel physically and emotionally. By cultivating this mindful approach to eating, you can develop a healthier relationship with food and nourish your body more effectively.

4. Engage Your Senses:

Use all your senses to fully experience your food. Notice the colors, shapes, smells, sounds, and tastes of each dish.

Engaging your senses while eating food involves using all of your senses—sight, smell, taste, touch, and even hearing—to fully experience and appreciate your meals. By bringing awareness to each sensory aspect of the food, you can enhance the enjoyment and satisfaction of eating.

Start by taking a moment to observe the appearance of your food—notice the colors, shapes, and presentation. Then, bring the food close to your nose and inhale deeply to appreciate its aroma. As you take a bite, pay attention to the texture and how it feels in your mouth. Chew slowly and savor the taste, allowing the flavors to fully develop on your palate.

You can also listen to the sounds of eating, such as the crunch of a fresh salad or the sizzle of food cooking on the stove, which can add another layer to the sensory experience.

Engaging your senses while eating can help you become more mindful and present during meals, leading to greater satisfaction and enjoyment of the food you consume.

5. Non-judgmental Awareness:

Practice observing your thoughts and emotions without judgment as you eat. Notice any cravings, distractions, or judgments that arise, and gently bring your focus back to the present moment.

Non-judgmental awareness while eating food involves observing your thoughts, emotions, and sensations related to eating without attaching judgment or criticism to them. It's about being fully present in the moment and accepting your experiences without labeling them as good or bad.

When practicing non-judgmental awareness, you may notice thoughts or emotions arise, such as cravings, guilt, or judgments about the food you're eating. Instead of reacting to these thoughts, simply acknowledge them and let them pass without getting caught up in them.

For example, if you find yourself feeling guilty about indulging in a dessert, instead of berating yourself for it, acknowledge the feeling with compassion and curiosity. Recognize that it's okay to enjoy treats occasionally and let go of any negative self-talk.

By cultivating non-judgmental awareness while eating, you can develop a healthier relationship with food and yourself. This practice encourages self-compassion, mindfulness, and a greater sense of peace and balance around eating habits.

6. Appreciation:

Cultivate gratitude for the nourishment and pleasure that food provides. Take a moment to appreciate the effort and care that went into preparing the meal.

Appreciation while eating food involves cultivating gratitude and recognition for the nourishment, flavors, and experiences that food provides. It's about approaching meals with a sense of mindfulness and acknowledging the effort and care that goes into preparing and enjoying food.

When you practice appreciation while eating, you take the time to truly savor and enjoy each bite, acknowledging the flavors, textures, and aromas of the food. You may also express gratitude for the individuals involved in bringing the food to your plate, such as farmers, cooks, or loved ones who prepared the meal.

By fostering a sense of appreciation while eating, you can develop a deeper connection to your food and a greater awareness of its impact on your well-being. This practice encourages mindful eating habits and can lead to increased satisfaction and enjoyment of meals.

Additionally, expressing gratitude for the food you consume can promote a more positive relationship with eating and foster a sense of abundance and contentment.

By incorporating these mindful eating techniques into your daily routine, you can develop a more mindful and balanced relationship with food, leading to greater enjoyment, satisfaction, and overall well-being.

3.3 Overcoming Emotional Eating

Overcoming emotional eating involves recognizing and addressing the underlying emotions and triggers that lead to overeating or using food as a coping mechanism. Emotional eating often occurs in response to stress, boredom, sadness, or other difficult emotions, and it can become a habitual response to managing emotional discomfort.

One approach to overcoming emotional eating is to cultivate greater self-awareness and mindfulness around eating habits. This involves paying attention to the thoughts, feelings, and physical sensations that arise before, during, and after eating. By identifying patterns and triggers associated with emotional eating, individuals can begin to develop alternative coping strategies for dealing with their emotions.

Another important aspect of overcoming emotional eating is learning to differentiate between physical hunger and emotional hunger. Physical hunger typically develops gradually and is accompanied by physical sensations such as stomach growling or low energy levels. Emotional hunger, on the other hand, tends to be sudden and intense and is often accompanied by cravings for specific types of foods.

Developing healthy coping mechanisms for managing emotions is essential for overcoming emotional eating. This may involve finding alternative ways to deal with stress or negative emotions, such as practicing relaxation techniques, engaging in physical activity, or seeking support from friends, family, or a therapist.

It's also important to cultivate a positive relationship with food and to practice self-care and self-compassion. This may involve learning to enjoy food without guilt or judgment, honoring hunger and fullness cues, and focusing on nourishing the body with balanced and nutritious meals.

By addressing the underlying emotional triggers and developing healthier coping mechanisms, individuals can gradually overcome emotional eating and develop a more balanced and mindful approach to eating and self-care.

Chapter 4: Exercise and Movement

Exercise and movement are essential components of a healthy lifestyle, contributing to physical fitness, mental well-being, and overall quality of life.

Exercise refers to planned, structured physical activity with the specific goal of improving fitness or health, while movement encompasses any form of bodily activity, including daily activities like walking, gardening, or taking the stairs.

Regular exercise offers a multitude of benefits for both physical and mental health. It helps to strengthen muscles and bones, improve cardiovascular health, and enhance flexibility and mobility.

Exercise also plays a crucial role in managing weight, reducing the risk of chronic diseases such as heart disease, diabetes, and certain cancers, and improving overall longevity.

In addition to its physical benefits, exercise has profound effects on mental health and well-being. It has been shown to reduce symptoms of anxiety and depression, improve mood, boost self-esteem, and enhance cognitive function.

Engaging in regular physical activity can also provide a sense of accomplishment and mastery, leading to increased feelings of happiness and fulfillment.

Movement, on the other hand, refers to any form of physical activity that gets the body moving. This includes activities like walking, dancing, stretching, and even fidgeting.

Incorporating more movement into daily life can have significant health benefits, such as reducing the risk of sedentary-related health problems like obesity and metabolic syndrome.

Whether through structured exercise routines or simply by incorporating more movement into daily activities, prioritizing physical activity is key to maintaining optimal health and well-being. Finding activities that are enjoyable and sustainable is essential for creating a long-term exercise routine that supports overall health and vitality.

4.1 Benefits of Physical Activity

Physical activity offers numerous benefits for both physical and mental health. Firstly, it contributes to overall physical fitness by improving cardiovascular health, increasing muscle strength and endurance, enhancing flexibility and balance, and promoting healthy weight management.

Regular physical activity can also reduce the risk of developing chronic diseases such as heart disease, type 2 diabetes, and certain types of cancer. Moreover, engaging in regular physical activity is crucial for maintaining bone health and reducing the risk of osteoporosis, particularly as individuals age.

Physical activity helps to stimulate bone growth and strengthen bones, which can help prevent fractures and maintain overall bone density. Beyond its physical benefits, physical activity also has profound effects on mental well-being.

Exercise has been shown to reduce symptoms of anxiety and depression, improve mood, boost self-esteem, and enhance cognitive function. It can also provide a sense of accomplishment and purpose, leading to increased feelings of happiness and fulfillment.

Furthermore, regular physical activity can improve sleep quality, reduce stress levels, and increase energy levels, ultimately leading to a better overall quality of life. Overall, incorporating regular physical activity into one's routine is essential for promoting health, vitality, and well-being across all aspects of life.

4.2 Finding Your Exercise Routine

Finding your exercise routine involves exploring different types of physical activities to discover what works best for your body, preferences, and lifestyle. Here are some steps to help you find an exercise routine that suits you:

1. Identify Your Goals:

Determine what you want to achieve through exercise, whether it's improving fitness, losing weight, reducing stress, or increasing energy levels.

Identifying your goals is a crucial first step in establishing an effective exercise routine tailored to your needs and aspirations. Your goals serve as a guiding force, helping you stay focused, motivated, and accountable throughout your fitness journey. Here's how to identify your exercise goals:

1. Determine Your Objectives:

    Reflect on what you hope to achieve through exercise. Whether it's improving overall health, losing weight, building muscle, increasing flexibility, reducing stress, or enhancing athletic performance, clarifying your objectives will shape your exercise routine.
2. Prioritize Your Goals:
    Consider which goals are most important to you and which ones you want to prioritize in your exercise routine. You may have multiple objectives, but it's helpful to identify the primary goals that will drive your fitness efforts.
3. Make Your Goals Specific and Measurable:

    Ensure that your goals are clear, specific, and measurable. Instead of saying you want to "get fit," specify that you aim to run a 5K race in under 30 minutes or to increase your strength by lifting a certain weight.

4. Set Realistic and Achievable Targets:
    Set goals that are challenging yet attainable within a reasonable timeframe. Setting unrealistic expectations can lead to frustration and demotivation. Break down larger goals into smaller, manageable milestones to track your progress effectively.
5. Consider Your Lifestyle and Preferences:
    Take into account your lifestyle, schedule, and personal preferences when setting exercise goals. Choose activities that you enjoy and that align with your interests and available time commitments.

By clearly identifying your exercise goals, you can design a tailored fitness plan that aligns with your objectives, maximizes your motivation, and ultimately leads to success in achieving your desired outcomes.

2. Assess Your Preferences:

Consider the types of activities you enjoy, whether it's swimming, cycling, dancing, yoga, or team sports. Choosing activities you like increases the likelihood of sticking with your routine.

Assessing your preferences is an essential step in creating an exercise routine that you will enjoy and stick with in the long term. Understanding what types of activities resonate with you ensures that your fitness regimen aligns with your interests, making it more likely for you to stay motivated and committed. Here's how to assess your exercise preferences:

1. Reflect on Past Experiences:
   Consider any physical activities or sports you have enjoyed in the past. Reflect on what aspects of those activities you found most enjoyable, whether it was the sense of accomplishment, the social aspect, or the physical challenge.
2. Identify Your Interests:
   Think about the types of activities that appeal to you. Do you enjoy outdoor activities like hiking or cycling, or do you prefer indoor activities like yoga or dancing? Consider whether you prefer individual activities or group settings.
3. Consider Your Personality:
   Take into account your personality traits and preferences. If you're competitive, you might enjoy team sports or group fitness classes. If you value solitude and introspection, activities like running or swimming might be more appealing.
4. Assess Accessibility and Convenience:
   Evaluate the availability of different exercise options in your area and consider factors such as cost, location, and scheduling. Choose activities that are easily accessible and fit into your lifestyle.
5. Experiment and Explore:
   Don't be afraid to try out different types of activities to see what resonates with you. Experiment with a variety of exercises, classes, or sports until you find the ones that you genuinely enjoy and look forward to.

By assessing your preferences thoughtfully, you can design an exercise routine that is enjoyable, sustainable, and tailored to your unique interests and lifestyle. This increases the likelihood of sticking with your fitness regimen and achieving your health and wellness goals.

Start Slowly:

Begin with activities that are manageable and enjoyable for your current fitness level. Gradually increase the intensity and duration of your workouts as your fitness improves.

Starting slowly is a prudent approach when beginning an exercise routine, especially if you are new to physical activity or returning after a period of inactivity. Taking gradual steps allows your body to adapt to increased demands, reducing the risk of injury and helping you build a strong foundation for long-term success. Here's why starting slowly is important:

Prevents Injury:

Beginning with low-intensity workouts allows your muscles, joints, and connective tissues to adapt gradually to the demands of exercise. This reduces the risk of strains, sprains, and other injuries commonly associated with overexertion.

Builds Confidence:

Starting slowly enables you to build confidence in your abilities and gradually increase your comfort level with exercise. Success with manageable workouts boosts self-esteem and motivation, making it more likely for you to stick with your routine over time.

Establishes Consistency:

Consistency is key to achieving your fitness goals. Starting slowly helps you establish a consistent exercise habit without overwhelming yourself. It sets a sustainable pace that you can maintain in the long run.

Allows for Progression:

By starting with manageable workouts, you create room for progression as your fitness improves. You can gradually increase the intensity, duration, or frequency of your workouts over time, challenging your body in a controlled manner.

Enhances Enjoyment:

Starting slowly allows you to focus on the enjoyment and benefits of exercise without feeling overwhelmed or discouraged. It enables you to discover activities you genuinely enjoy and develop a positive relationship with physical activity.

Whether it's beginning with shorter workout sessions, lower resistance levels, or slower-paced activities, starting slowly sets the stage for a safe, enjoyable, and sustainable exercise journey. It's a valuable investment in your long-term health and well-being.

Mix It Up:

Incorporate a variety of activities into your routine to keep things interesting and prevent boredom. This could include cardio, strength training, flexibility exercises, and activities that promote balance and coordination.

Mixing up your exercise routine involves incorporating a variety of activities and workouts to keep your workouts interesting, challenging, and effective. This approach offers numerous benefits for both physical and mental health, as well as helping to prevent boredom and plateaus. Here's why mixing up your exercise routine is important:

Prevents Boredom:

Variety keeps workouts fresh and exciting, preventing boredom and monotony. Trying new activities and exercises can make exercise more enjoyable and engaging, motivating you to stick with your routine.

Targets Different Muscle Groups:

Incorporating a variety of exercises targets different muscle groups, helping to improve overall strength, endurance, and flexibility. This balanced approach ensures that all areas of the body are adequately trained and reduces the risk of overuse injuries.

Maximizes Results:

Mixing up your workouts challenges your body in new ways, helping to break through plateaus and maximize results. By constantly challenging yourself with different exercises and intensities, you can continue to make progress towards your fitness goals.

Reduces Risk of Burnout:

Repeating the same workout routine day after day can lead to burnout and decreased motivation. Mixing up your exercise routine allows for greater flexibility and adaptability, reducing the likelihood of burnout and keeping you motivated in the long term.

Offers Mental Stimulation:

Trying new activities and learning new skills provides mental stimulation and can improve cognitive function. Mixing up your exercise routine keeps your mind engaged and focused, enhancing the overall experience of exercise.

Incorporating a variety of activities, such as cardio, strength training, flexibility exercises, and recreational sports, ensures a well-rounded fitness regimen that promotes overall health and well-being. Whether it's trying a new fitness class, exploring outdoor activities, or incorporating bodyweight exercises into your routine, mixing up your exercise regimen keeps workouts fun, challenging, and effective.

Listen to Your Body:

Pay attention to how your body feels during and after exercise. Choose activities that make you feel good physically and mentally, and be mindful of any discomfort or pain that may indicate the need to adjust your routine.

Listening to your body is an essential aspect of any exercise routine, as it allows you to respond to your body's needs and signals, ultimately promoting safety, effectiveness, and overall well-being. Here's why listening to your body is crucial:

1. Prevents Injury:
   Paying attention to how your body feels during exercise helps you avoid pushing yourself too hard or ignoring warning signs of potential injury. Tuning into sensations of discomfort or pain allows you to adjust your workout intensity or technique to prevent overexertion or strain.

2. Honors Your Limits:
   Every individual has unique physical capabilities and limitations. Listening to your body enables you to respect and honor your limits, rather than pushing past them unnecessarily. Recognizing when you need to take a break or modify an exercise helps prevent burnout and promotes a sustainable approach to fitness.

3. Indicates Recovery Needs:
   Your body provides valuable feedback about its recovery needs after exercise. Sensations of fatigue, soreness, or stiffness signal that your muscles need time to repair and rebuild. Listening to your body's cues allows you to incorporate adequate rest and recovery into your routine, preventing overtraining and promoting optimal performance.

4. Guides Nutrition and Hydration:
   Proper nutrition and hydration are essential for supporting exercise performance and recovery. Listening to your body's hunger and thirst signals helps ensure that you fuel and hydrate appropriately before, during, and after workouts. This promotes energy levels, enhances performance, and supports muscle repair and recovery.

5. Promotes Mindfulness and Self-Awareness:
   Listening to your body fosters mindfulness and self-awareness, allowing you to develop a deeper connection with your body and its needs. This heightened awareness extends beyond exercise and can positively impact other areas of your life, promoting holistic well-being.

Overall, listening to your body is a fundamental principle of safe and effective exercise. By tuning into your body's signals and responding with care and respect, you can optimize your workouts, prevent injury, and promote overall health and vitality.

Set Realistic Expectations:

Be patient and realistic about your progress. Results may take time, so focus on consistency and making exercise a regular part of your routine.

Setting realistic expectations is crucial when embarking on an exercise journey, as it helps you maintain motivation, prevent disappointment, and achieve sustainable progress towards your fitness goals. Here's why setting realistic expectations is essential:

1. Promotes Long-Term Success:
   Realistic expectations set the foundation for long-term success by acknowledging that progress takes time and effort. By setting achievable goals and recognizing that change won't happen overnight, you're more likely to stay committed to your exercise routine and see gradual improvements over time.
2. Prevents Frustration and Disappointment:
   Unrealistic expectations can lead to frustration and disappointment when you don't see immediate results or meet lofty goals. Setting realistic expectations helps manage your emotions and maintain a positive mindset, even in the face of challenges or setbacks.
3. Encourages Sustainable Habits:
   Realistic expectations encourage the development of sustainable exercise habits by focusing on gradual progress and consistency rather than quick fixes or extreme measures. By adopting realistic goals that align with your abilities and lifestyle, you're more likely to establish healthy habits that you can maintain in the long run.
4. Celebrates Achievements:
   Setting realistic expectations allows you to celebrate achievements, no matter how small. By recognizing and acknowledging your progress along the way, you stay motivated and inspired to continue working towards your goals.
5. Enhances Self-Efficacy:
   Realistic expectations build confidence and self-efficacy by demonstrating that you have the ability to make meaningful changes and achieve your goals through effort and perseverance. This positive reinforcement strengthens your belief in your capabilities and empowers you to overcome obstacles and setbacks.

Overall, setting realistic expectations is essential for fostering a positive and sustainable approach to exercise. By embracing gradual progress, celebrating achievements, and staying committed to your goals, you can create a fulfilling and rewarding exercise journey that supports your long-term health and well-being.

By experimenting with different activities and listening to your body's feedback, you can create an exercise routine that is enjoyable, effective, and sustainable for the long term.

4.3 Incorporating Movement In to Daily Life

Incorporating movement into daily life is essential for maintaining overall health, vitality, and well-being. By finding opportunities to be active throughout the day, you can increase physical activity levels, reduce sedentary behavior, and reap numerous health benefits. Here are some ways to incorporate movement into your daily routine:

1. Take the Stairs:
   Opt for stairs instead of elevators or escalators whenever possible. Climbing stairs is an excellent way to increase heart rate, build leg strength, and burn calories.
2. Walk or Bike:
   Whenever feasible, walk or bike instead of driving for short distances. This not only adds physical activity to your day but also reduces carbon emissions and promotes environmental sustainability.
3. Stand Up and Move:
   Break up long periods of sitting by standing up and moving around regularly. Set a timer to remind yourself to stretch, take a short walk, or do some light exercises every hour.
4. Do Household Chores:
   Turn household chores into opportunities for physical activity. Vacuuming, gardening, mopping, and cleaning can all provide a decent workout and contribute to daily movement goals.
5. Take Active Breaks:
   Instead of sitting during breaks at work or while watching TV, take active breaks. Stand up, stretch, do some squats or lunges, or go for a quick walk to refresh your mind and body.
6. Engage in Active Hobbies:
   Choose hobbies and recreational activities that involve movement, such as dancing, swimming, hiking, or playing sports. Not only do these activities provide physical benefits, but they also promote enjoyment and social interaction.
7. Park Farther Away:

Park your car farther away from your destination to add extra steps to your day. Walking a few extra minutes can accumulate significant physical activity over time.

By incorporating movement into your daily life, you can improve your overall health, increase energy levels, reduce the risk of chronic diseases, and enhance your quality of life. Making small changes to prioritize physical activity throughout the day can lead to significant long-term benefits for both body and mind.

Chapter 5: Building Healthy Habits

Building healthy habits is essential for achieving and maintaining overall well-being and longevity. These habits not only improve physical health but also contribute to mental, emotional, and social well-being. Here's how to build healthy habits:

Building healthy habits is essential for maintaining physical, mental, and emotional well-being. It involves adopting behaviors that promote overall health and vitality while gradually eliminating harmful practices. One key aspect of cultivating healthy habits is consistency. Whether it's regular exercise, balanced nutrition, or sufficient sleep, making these activities a regular part of your routine is crucial.

Another important component is setting realistic goals. Breaking down larger objectives into smaller, achievable steps can make the process more manageable and sustainable. Additionally, staying mindful and aware of your habits allows you to track progress and make adjustments as needed.

Building a support system can also enhance success in developing healthy habits. Surrounding yourself with people who encourage and motivate you can provide accountability and inspiration.

Ultimately, building healthy habits is a journey that requires commitment, patience, and self-awareness. By prioritizing your well-being and taking proactive steps towards positive change, you can cultivate a lifestyle that fosters long-term health and happiness.

1. Start Small:

    Begin by making small, manageable changes to your daily routine. Choose one or two specific habits to focus on at a time, such as drinking more water, eating more fruits and vegetables, or getting regular exercise.

    Starting small is a powerful strategy when building healthy habits as it allows you to gradually integrate positive changes into your lifestyle. By focusing on small, achievable steps, you set yourself up for success and avoid feeling overwhelmed. Here's why starting small is effective:

    1. Manageable Changes:

        Starting with small changes makes them more manageable and less intimidating. It's easier to incorporate minor adjustments into your routine, such as drinking an extra glass of water each day or adding a serving of vegetables to your meals.

    2. Establishes a Foundation:

        Small changes serve as the foundation for larger, more significant habits over time. By mastering smaller habits first, you build confidence and momentum, making it easier to tackle more ambitious goals in the future.

    3. Increases Success Rate:

        Starting small increases your likelihood of success. Achieving small victories boosts motivation and reinforces the belief that you can make positive changes, paving the way for continued progress.

4. Creates Lasting Change:
   Building habits is about consistency and repetition. Starting small allows you to establish a solid foundation of consistent behavior, making it easier to maintain healthy habits over the long term.

5. Builds Confidence:
   Each small success builds confidence and reinforces your ability to make positive changes. Over time, this increased confidence empowers you to tackle more challenging habits and make lasting improvements to your health and well-being.

By starting small and gradually building on your successes, you can create sustainable, long-lasting healthy habits that contribute to a healthier and happier lifestyle.

Set Realistic Goals:

Set achievable and realistic goals that are specific, measurable, and time-bound. Break larger goals into smaller, actionable steps to make progress more manageable and attainable.

Setting realistic goals is essential for building healthy habits that are sustainable and achievable. Realistic goals provide a clear roadmap for success and help you stay motivated throughout your journey. Here's why setting realistic goals is important:

1. Achievability:
   Realistic goals are attainable within your current abilities, resources, and circumstances. They take into account factors such as time, energy, and commitment, making them feasible to accomplish.

2. Motivation:
   Realistic goals provide a sense of purpose and direction, motivating you to take action and stay focused on your objectives. Achieving smaller milestones along the way boosts confidence and momentum, fueling your motivation to continue working towards your larger goals.

3. Accountability:
   Realistic goals help hold you accountable for your progress. By setting specific and measurable targets, you can track your achievements and identify areas where adjustments may be needed to stay on track.

4. Sustainability:
   Realistic goals promote sustainable behavior change by setting a pace that is manageable and maintainable over the long term. They encourage gradual progress and allow for flexibility in adapting to challenges and setbacks.

5. Positive Reinforcement:
   Meeting realistic goals reinforces positive behaviors and builds self-confidence. Celebrating small victories along the way reinforces your commitment to your goals and strengthens your belief in your ability to achieve them.

Overall, setting realistic goals sets the stage for success by providing a clear roadmap, maintaining motivation, and fostering sustainable behavior change. By establishing achievable targets that align with your capabilities and priorities, you can build healthy habits that endure and contribute to lasting well-being.

Be Consistent:

Consistency is key to building habits. Incorporate your chosen habits into your daily routine and make them a priority. Aim to practice your habits consistently, even on days when you feel less motivated or busy.

Consistency is key when it comes to building healthy habits and achieving your goals. By maintaining a regular and steady effort over time, you can make meaningful progress and create lasting changes in your life. Here's why consistency is important:

1. Establishes Routine:
   Consistency helps you establish a routine by making healthy habits a regular part of your daily life. By consistently practicing these habits, they become ingrained behaviors that require less effort and willpower to maintain.

2. Builds Momentum:
   Consistent effort builds momentum and propels you forward towards your goals. Each small step taken consistently adds up over time, leading to significant progress and results.

3. Reinforces Behavior:
   Consistency reinforces positive behavior by creating neural pathways in the brain associated with the habit. The more frequently you engage in a behavior, the stronger these neural connections become, making it easier to maintain the habit in the long run.

4. Overcomes Resistance:
   Consistency helps you overcome resistance and push through challenges or obstacles that may arise along the way. By committing to showing up and putting in the effort consistently, you build resilience and perseverance.

5. Creates Accountability:
   Consistency holds you accountable for your actions and progress. When you commit to being consistent, you're more likely to follow through on your intentions and take responsibility for your results.

6. Builds Trust:
   Consistency builds trust and reliability, both with yourself and with others. When you consistently follow through on your commitments and actions, you develop a reputation for dependability and integrity.

Achieves Long-Term Success:

Consistency is the key to long-term success. By consistently practicing healthy habits and staying committed to your goals, you set yourself up for sustainable progress and lasting change.

summary, consistency is essential for building healthy habits, achieving your goals, and creating positive change in your life. By staying committed and showing up consistently, you can unlock your full potential and create the life you desire.

2. Track Your Progress:

Keep track of your progress to stay motivated and accountable. Use a journal, app, or calendar to record your habits, track your successes, and identify areas for improvement.

Tracking your progress is a vital aspect of achieving your goals and maintaining motivation on your journey towards building healthy habits. By monitoring your progress, you gain valuable insights into your successes, areas for improvement, and overall growth. Here's why tracking your progress is important:

1. Provides Accountability:
   Tracking your progress holds you accountable for your actions and commitments. It helps you stay focused on your goals and motivates you to take consistent steps towards achieving them.

2. Measures Success:
   Tracking allows you to measure your success and see how far you've come since starting your journey. It provides tangible evidence of your progress, boosting confidence and reinforcing your belief in your ability to succeed.

3. Identifies Patterns:
   Monitoring your progress helps you identify patterns and trends in your behavior, habits, and outcomes. It allows you to recognize what strategies are working well and where adjustments may be needed to optimize results.

4. Celebrates Milestones:
   Tracking your progress enables you to celebrate milestones and achievements along the way. Recognizing and acknowledging your successes, no matter how small, boosts morale and keeps you motivated to continue working towards your goals.

5. Adjusts Strategies:
   By tracking your progress, you can assess the effectiveness of your current strategies and make informed decisions about what changes may be necessary. It allows you to pivot and adapt your approach as needed to overcome challenges and obstacles.

Provides Feedback:
Progress tracking provides valuable feedback that helps you learn and grow from your experiences. It allows you to reflect on what has worked well and what could be improved, guiding future actions and decisions.

6. Enhances Focus:
Tracking your progress keeps your goals at the forefront of your mind and enhances focus and clarity. It helps you prioritize tasks and activities that align with your objectives, reducing distractions and increasing productivity.

In summary, tracking your progress is essential for maintaining accountability, measuring success, identifying patterns, celebrating milestones, adjusting strategies, receiving feedback, and enhancing focus on your journey towards building healthy habits and achieving your goals.

Whether you use a journal, app, spreadsheet, or another method, regularly tracking your progress can significantly contribute to your overall success and well-being.

3. Stay Flexible:

Be flexible and adaptable in your approach to building healthy habits. Life can be unpredictable, and there may be times when you face challenges or setbacks. Instead of giving up, adjust your strategy and find alternative ways to stay on track.

Staying flexible is a crucial mindset when it comes to building healthy habits and achieving your goals. Flexibility allows you to adapt to changing circumstances, overcome obstacles, and continue making progress on your journey, even in the face of challenges. Here's why staying flexible is important:

1. Adapts to Changes:
Life is unpredictable, and unexpected changes are inevitable. Staying flexible enables you to adapt to new situations, environments, or circumstances that may arise, allowing you to continue working towards your goals despite disruptions.

2. Adjusts Strategies:
Not every plan or approach will work perfectly the first time. Staying flexible allows you to evaluate your strategies and make adjustments as needed. It empowers you to try new methods, experiment with different approaches, and find what works best for you.

3. Overcomes Setbacks:
Setbacks and obstacles are a natural part of any journey. Staying flexible helps you bounce back from setbacks and navigate challenges with resilience and determination. It enables you to learn from setbacks, refocus your efforts, and keep moving forward.

4. Maintains Motivation:
Rigidity can lead to frustration and burnout when things don't go as planned. Staying flexible helps maintain motivation by allowing you to stay open-minded, optimistic, and adaptable in the face of setbacks or unexpected circumstances.

5. Embraces Opportunities:
   Staying flexible opens you up to new opportunities and possibilities that may arise along the way. It allows you to seize opportunities for growth, learning, and personal development, even if they deviate from your original plan.

6. Reduces Stress:
   Flexibility reduces stress by promoting a more relaxed and adaptable mindset. Instead of resisting change or becoming overwhelmed by unexpected events, staying flexible enables you to approach challenges with a sense of calmness and acceptance.

7. Promotes Resilience:
   Ultimately, staying flexible promotes resilience, which is the ability to bounce back from adversity stronger and more resilient than before. By embracing flexibility, you build resilience muscles that help you overcome obstacles and thrive in the face of adversity.

In summary, staying flexible is essential for navigating life's twists and turns, overcoming obstacles, maintaining motivation, and ultimately achieving your goals. By cultivating a flexible mindset, you empower yourself to adapt, grow, and succeed in any situation that comes your way.

4. Find Support:
   Surround yourself with a supportive network of friends, family, or like-minded individuals who can encourage and motivate you on your journey. Share your goals and progress with others, and seek support when needed.

Finding support is an invaluable resource when it comes to building healthy habits and achieving your goals. Having a supportive network of friends, family, or like-minded individuals can provide encouragement, accountability, and motivation to help you stay on track and overcome challenges. Here's why finding support is important:

1. Encouragement:
   Supportive individuals offer encouragement and positive reinforcement, helping you stay motivated and focused on your goals. Their words of encouragement can provide a much-needed boost during times of doubt or difficulty.

2. Accountability:
   A supportive network holds you accountable for your actions and commitments. Knowing that others are rooting for you and expecting you to follow through on your goals can help you stay committed and responsible for your progress.

3. Motivation:
   Supportive individuals can serve as sources of inspiration and motivation, sharing their own successes, experiences, and tips for staying on track. Their encouragement and motivation can help you push through obstacles and stay motivated on your journey.

4. Emotional Support:
   Building healthy habits can be challenging, and it's normal to experience moments of frustration, self-doubt, or discouragement. Having a support system to lean on during

difficult times provides emotional support and reassurance, reminding you that you're not alone in your struggles.

5. Practical Assistance:
   Supportive individuals can offer practical assistance, whether it's helping you brainstorm solutions to obstacles, providing resources or information, or even participating in activities together. Their practical support can make it easier to overcome barriers and make progress towards your goals.

6. Celebrating Successes:
   Supportive individuals celebrate your successes and milestones with you, no matter how small. Sharing your achievements with others who genuinely care about your well-being reinforces your progress and boosts your confidence.

7. Sense of Belonging:
   Finding support creates a sense of belonging and connection to a community of individuals who share similar goals and values. Knowing that you're part of a supportive network can enhance your sense of purpose and belonging, fostering a supportive environment for growth and change.

In summary, finding support is essential for building healthy habits and achieving your goals. Whether it's friends, family, support groups, or online communities, surrounding yourself with supportive individuals can provide encouragement, accountability, motivation, and practical assistance to help you succeed on your journey towards health and well-being.

5. Practice Self-Compassion:

Be kind to yourself and practice self-compassion throughout the process of building healthy habits. Acknowledge your efforts and celebrate your successes, no matter how small. Treat yourself with kindness and understanding, especially during times of difficulty or setbacks.

Practicing self-compassion is a fundamental aspect of building healthy habits and fostering overall well-being. It involves treating oneself with kindness, understanding, and acceptance, especially during times of difficulty or setback. Here's why practicing self-compassion is important:

1. Reduces Self-Criticism:
   Self-compassion helps to counteract negative self-talk and self-criticism, which can undermine confidence and motivation. Instead of berating yourself for perceived shortcomings or mistakes, self-compassion encourages self-kindness and understanding.
2. Promotes Resilience:
   Self-compassion promotes resilience by providing a buffer against stress, setbacks, and failures. It allows you to respond to challenges with greater emotional resilience and bounce back more quickly from adversity.
3. Cultivates Positive Mindset:
   Practicing self-compassion cultivates a more positive mindset and fosters feelings of self-worth and self-esteem. By acknowledging your humanity and inherent value, you can approach life's challenges with greater optimism and confidence.
4. Enhances Motivation:

Self-compassion enhances motivation by fostering a supportive and nurturing inner dialogue. Rather than relying on harsh self-criticism to drive change, self-compassion motivates you through encouragement, self-care, and a focus on growth and improvement.

5. Encourages Self-Care:

    Self-compassion encourages self-care and prioritizing your own well-being. It involves tuning into your needs, practicing self-kindness, and engaging in activities that promote physical, emotional, and mental health.

6. Strengthens Relationships:

    Practicing self-compassion can improve relationships with others by fostering empathy, understanding, and acceptance. When you treat yourself with kindness and compassion, you're better able to extend those qualities to others, leading to more fulfilling and supportive relationships.

    Fosters Emotional Healing:

    Self-compassion facilitates emotional healing by allowing you to process difficult emotions with greater gentleness and acceptance. It creates a safe space for acknowledging and validating your feelings, leading to greater emotional resilience and well-being.

In summary, practicing self-compassion is essential for building healthy habits, fostering resilience, enhancing motivation, and promoting overall well-being. By treating yourself with kindness, understanding, and acceptance, you can cultivate a more positive relationship with yourself and navigate life's challenges with greater ease and grace.

By following these steps and incorporating healthy habits into your daily life, you can create positive, sustainable changes that promote long-term health and well-being. Remember that building healthy habits is a journey, and progress takes time, patience, and dedication.

5.1   The Power of Habits

The power of habits lies in their ability to shape our actions, behaviors, and ultimately, our lives. Habits are automatic routines and behaviors that we perform regularly, often without conscious thought.

They have a profound impact on our daily lives, influencing everything from our health and productivity to our relationships and success. Here's why understanding and harnessing the power of habits is important:

1. Creates Consistency:

    Habits provide structure and consistency to our lives by establishing regular routines and behaviors. Consistent habits help us stay organized, manage our time effectively, and achieve our goals more efficiently.

    Creating consistency is essential for achieving success in any endeavor, whether it be personal or professional. Consistency is the habit of continuously showing up and putting in the effort, even when it's challenging or when immediate results aren't apparent.

It's about developing routines, sticking to schedules, and maintaining a steadfast commitment to your goals.

Consistency breeds reliability and builds trust, both with yourself and with others. When you consistently deliver on your promises and meet expectations, you establish yourself as someone dependable and worthy of respect.

This reliability forms the foundation of strong relationships, whether they're with colleagues, clients, friends, or family.

Consistency also plays a crucial role in skill development and improvement. By consistently practicing and honing your skills, you gradually progress and become more proficient in your craft. Whether it's learning a new language, mastering a musical instrument, or excelling in a sport, the key to improvement lies in regular, consistent effort over time.

Moreover, consistency helps to maintain momentum and overcome obstacles. When faced with challenges or setbacks, it's the consistency of your efforts that keeps you moving forward. By staying committed to your goals and persevering through difficulties, you build resilience and develop the perseverance necessary to overcome any obstacles that come your way.

In summary, creating consistency is about establishing habits, routines, and behaviors that align with your goals and values. It's about showing up consistently, putting in the effort, and staying committed, even when the going gets tough. By doing so, you lay the groundwork for success, build trust and reliability, and ultimately, achieve your desired outcomes.

1. Shapes Behavior:

    Habits play a significant role in shaping our behavior and decision-making processes. Positive habits, such as exercising regularly or practicing mindfulness, lead to healthier choices and outcomes, while negative habits can undermine our well-being and success.

    Shaping behavior involves using various strategies to encourage or discourage certain actions, habits, or responses in individuals. It's a fundamental concept in psychology and is widely used in fields such as education, parenting, therapy, and organizational management.

    One of the most common methods of shaping behavior is through positive reinforcement. This involves rewarding desired behaviors to increase the likelihood of them occurring again in the future. For example, praising a student for completing their homework on time can reinforce the behavior of timely completion.

    Another strategy is negative reinforcement, which involves removing or avoiding negative consequences to encourage desired behaviors. An example of this would be allowing an employee to leave work early if they consistently meet their targets, thereby reinforcing their productivity.

Additionally, shaping behavior can involve using punishment, although this strategy is generally less effective in the long term and can have negative side effects such as resentment or avoidance. Instead, focusing on positive reinforcement and creating a supportive environment tends to yield better results.

Consistency is key when shaping behavior, as it helps reinforce the association between the behavior and its consequences. By consistently rewarding desired behaviors and providing feedback, individuals are more likely to understand what is expected of them and to adjust their actions accordingly.

Overall, shaping behavior is a powerful tool for influencing individual and group dynamics, promoting personal development, and fostering positive outcomes in various settings. Through understanding the principles of behavior shaping and applying them effectively, individuals and organizations can achieve their goals and cultivate healthier, more productive environments.

2. Saves Mental Energy:

Habits automate repetitive tasks and behaviors, freeing up mental energy for more complex decision-making and problem-solving. By making certain behaviors automatic, habits reduce cognitive load and help streamline daily routines.

Saving mental energy is crucial for maintaining cognitive functioning, productivity, and overall well-being. Mental energy refers to the capacity to focus, make decisions, and manage emotions effectively. Conserving mental energy involves adopting strategies to minimize unnecessary stress, distractions, and cognitive load.

One way to save mental energy is by establishing routines and habits. By automating repetitive tasks and decisions, such as setting a morning routine or meal planning, you free up mental bandwidth for more important activities. Routines provide structure and reduce the need for constant decision-making, thereby conserving mental energy.

Another effective strategy is prioritizing tasks and breaking them down into manageable chunks. By focusing on the most important or time-sensitive tasks first, you allocate your mental resources more efficiently. Breaking tasks into smaller steps also makes them less overwhelming, reducing mental strain and increasing productivity.

Limiting distractions is also essential for saving mental energy. This can involve setting boundaries with technology, such as turning off notifications or scheduling dedicated work periods without interruptions. Creating a conducive environment for focus helps minimize cognitive load and prevents mental fatigue.

Practicing mindfulness and stress-reduction techniques can also conserve mental energy. Activities such as meditation, deep breathing exercises, or taking short breaks throughout the day can help recharge your mental batteries and improve cognitive resilience.

Overall, saving mental energy requires a combination of proactive strategies, self-awareness, and intentional habits. By prioritizing tasks, minimizing distractions, and practicing self-care, you can optimize your cognitive resources and enhance your overall productivity and well-being.

3. Builds Momentum:

Habits create momentum and inertia, making it easier to maintain positive behaviors over time. Once established, habits require less effort and willpower to maintain, allowing us to sustain progress towards our goals with less resistance.

Building momentum is essential for achieving goals and making progress in any endeavor. Momentum refers to the force or energy gained by a moving object or by a series of successful actions. When applied to personal or professional development, momentum involves creating a positive cycle of progress and motivation that propels you forward.

One way momentum is built is by starting with small, achievable tasks and gradually increasing the level of challenge or complexity. By experiencing success with manageable goals, you build confidence and momentum to tackle more significant objectives.

Consistency is another key factor in building momentum. By consistently showing up and putting in the effort, you create a sense of rhythm and progress that keeps you moving forward. Small, consistent actions compound over time, leading to significant results.

Celebrating victories, no matter how small, is also crucial for maintaining momentum. Recognizing and acknowledging your progress reinforces positive behaviors and motivates you to continue pushing forward.

Additionally, surrounding yourself with supportive people and resources can help sustain momentum. Whether it's through accountability partners, mentors, or helpful tools and resources, having a support system in place can provide encouragement and guidance during challenging times.

Overall, building momentum is about taking consistent action, celebrating progress, and staying focused on your goals. By cultivating a positive cycle of success and motivation, you can overcome obstacles and achieve lasting results in any area of your life.

4. Supports Goal Achievement:

Habits are powerful tools for achieving long-term goals. By aligning our habits with our objectives, we can create a supportive environment that facilitates progress and success. Consistently practicing habits that reinforce our goals increases the likelihood of achieving them.

Supporting goal achievement involves implementing strategies and practices that facilitate progress towards desired objectives. It encompasses a range of actions and behaviors aimed at overcoming obstacles, staying motivated, and maintaining focus on the end goal.

Setting clear and specific goals is the first step in supporting goal achievement. By defining what you want to accomplish and breaking it down into manageable steps, you create a roadmap for success and increase clarity and direction.

Developing a plan of action is essential for translating goals into tangible results. This involves outlining the necessary tasks, deadlines, and resources needed to accomplish each step along the way. Having a structured plan provides guidance and helps maintain momentum towards goal attainment.

Seeking support from others can significantly aid in goal achievement. Whether it's through mentorship, collaboration, or accountability partnerships, involving others in your journey provides encouragement, feedback, and motivation to stay on track.

Monitoring progress and adjusting strategies as needed is crucial for overcoming challenges and staying adaptable. Regularly reviewing your progress allows you to identify areas for improvement and make necessary adjustments to ensure continued progress towards your goals.

Finally, celebrating milestones and successes along the way reinforces positive behaviors and keeps you motivated to pursue your goals. Recognizing and acknowledging your achievements provides a sense of accomplishment and fuels your drive to keep pushing forward.

In summary, supporting goal achievement involves setting clear goals, developing a plan of action, seeking support from others, monitoring progress, and celebrating successes. By implementing these strategies, you can overcome obstacles and achieve your desired outcomes effectively and efficiently.

5. Shapes Identity:

Habits shape our sense of identity and self-perception. The behaviors we repeatedly engage in become ingrained aspects of our identity, influencing how we see ourselves and how others perceive us.

Shaping identity involves the complex interplay of internal and external factors that contribute to the formation of an individual's sense of self. Identity encompasses various aspects, including personal values, beliefs, interests, cultural background, and experiences, all of which shape how individuals perceive themselves and how they are perceived by others.

One significant factor in shaping identity is socialization, which refers to the process through which individuals learn and internalize cultural norms, values, and expectations. Family, peers, schools, media, and other social institutions play crucial roles in shaping identity by providing models, feedback, and reinforcement of certain behaviors and beliefs.

Cultural influences also play a significant role in shaping identity. Individuals often identify with specific cultural groups based on shared values, traditions, language, and heritage. These cultural affiliations contribute to a sense of belonging and help shape how individuals perceive themselves within the broader context of society.

Personal experiences, including successes, failures, challenges, and triumphs, also play a vital role in shaping identity. These experiences shape individuals' beliefs about themselves, their capabilities, and their place in the world, ultimately influencing their sense of self-esteem, self-efficacy, and identity.

Additionally, self-reflection and introspection play a crucial role in identity formation. By examining their values, beliefs, and experiences, individuals can gain insight into their identity and make conscious choices about who they want to be.

In summary, shaping identity is a dynamic and multifaceted process influenced by social, cultural, and personal factors. It involves the internalization of beliefs, values, and experiences that contribute to an individual's sense of self and their place in the world.

6. Enables Personal Growth:

Understanding the power of habits empowers us to intentionally cultivate positive behaviors and break free from negative patterns. By harnessing the power of habits, we can create meaningful change in our lives, foster personal growth, and unlock our full potential.

Enabling personal growth involves fostering an environment and mindset conducive to self-improvement, learning, and development. It encompasses a range of actions and practices aimed at expanding one's capabilities, understanding, and fulfillment in various aspects of life.

One key aspect of enabling personal growth is cultivating a growth mindset. This mindset, as proposed by psychologist Carol Dweck, involves embracing challenges, persisting in the face of setbacks, and seeing failures as opportunities for learning and growth. By adopting a growth mindset, individuals are more likely to seek out new experiences, take risks, and continuously strive for self-improvement.

Setting and pursuing meaningful goals is another essential component of personal growth. By identifying areas for improvement and setting clear objectives, individuals can focus their efforts and energy on specific outcomes that contribute to their overall development and fulfillment.

Seeking feedback and guidance from others is also crucial for personal growth. Whether through mentorship, coaching, or constructive criticism, receiving input from others can provide valuable insights, perspective, and support for self-improvement.

Engaging in continuous learning and self-reflection is fundamental to personal growth. By seeking out new knowledge, skills, and experiences, individuals can expand their understanding of themselves and the world around them, fostering personal and intellectual growth.

Moreover, practicing self-care and prioritizing well-being are essential for enabling personal growth. Taking care of physical, emotional, and mental health allows individuals to maintain the resilience and energy needed to pursue their goals and thrive in various areas of life.

In summary, enabling personal growth involves fostering a growth mindset, setting meaningful goals, seeking feedback and guidance, engaging in continuous learning and self-reflection, and prioritizing well-being. By cultivating these habits and practices, individuals can unlock their full potential and experience ongoing growth and fulfillment in their lives.

In summary, the power of habits lies in their ability to create consistency, shape behavior, save mental energy, build momentum, support goal achievement, shape identity, and enable personal growth. By understanding how habits work and intentionally cultivating positive behaviors, we can harness their power to create a happier, healthier, and more fulfilling life.

5.2 Strategies for Building Healthy Habits

Building healthy habits is essential for maintaining overall well-being and achieving long-term success in various aspects of life. Here are some effective strategies for establishing and sustaining healthy habits:

1. Start Small:

   Begin by focusing on one or two manageable habits at a time. Trying to make too many changes at once can be overwhelming and unsustainable. For example, start with drinking more water each day or incorporating a short daily walk into your routine.

   Starting small is a powerful strategy for building healthy habits as it makes the process more manageable and increases the likelihood of success. By focusing on small, achievable actions, individuals can gradually incorporate healthier behaviors into their daily routines.

   One effective approach is to identify a specific habit you want to develop and break it down into smaller, more manageable steps. For example, if your goal is to eat more fruits and vegetables, you could start by adding one serving of a fruit or vegetable to one meal each day.

   Another strategy is to implement the "two-minute rule," which involves breaking down habits into tasks that can be completed in just two minutes. For instance, if your goal is to exercise more, commit to doing just two minutes of exercise each day, such as a quick walk around the block or a set of push-ups.

   Additionally, pairing new habits with existing ones can help reinforce them and make them easier to adopt. For example, if you want to start flossing your teeth regularly, you could pair it with brushing your teeth as part of your bedtime routine.

Overall, starting small allows individuals to build momentum, gain confidence, and gradually increase the complexity of their habits over time. By taking small, consistent steps, individuals can create lasting changes that contribute to their overall health and well-being.

2. Set Specific Goals:

Clearly define what you want to achieve with each habit. Make your goals measurable and realistic. Instead of saying "I want to exercise more," specify "I will go for a 30-minute walk three times a week."

Setting specific goals is a crucial strategy for building healthy habits as it provides clarity, motivation, and direction. Specific goals help individuals identify exactly what they want to achieve and outline the steps needed to reach them.

One effective approach is to use the SMART criteria when setting goals: Specific, Measurable, Achievable, Relevant, and Time-bound. This means defining your goals in clear and precise terms, such as "I will drink eight glasses of water every day" rather than a vague goal like "I will drink more water."

Additionally, breaking larger goals into smaller, more manageable milestones can make them less daunting and easier to achieve. For example, if your ultimate goal is to lose 20 pounds, you could set smaller monthly goals to lose 2-3 pounds each month.

Regularly reviewing and adjusting your goals as needed is also essential for staying on track and maintaining motivation. If you find that a particular goal is too challenging or not aligned with your priorities, don't hesitate to modify it accordingly.

By setting specific, achievable goals, individuals can create a roadmap for success and stay focused on making progress towards building healthy habits. Having clear goals provides a sense of purpose and direction, making it easier to stay motivated and committed to making positive changes in your life.

3. Create a Routine:

Establishing a consistent routine helps reinforce habits and make them automatic. Incorporate your new habit into your daily schedule at a specific time or trigger. For example, if you want to start meditating, designate a quiet time and place each day for your practice.

Creating a routine is a powerful strategy for building healthy habits as it provides structure, consistency, and accountability. Establishing a regular schedule helps individuals integrate healthy behaviors into their daily lives and make them a natural part of their routine.

One effective approach is to identify specific times of day for engaging in healthy habits and incorporating them into your daily schedule. For example, you could designate a morning routine that includes activities such as exercise, meditation, and healthy breakfast preparation.

Consistency is key when creating a routine, so it's essential to stick to your schedule as much as possible. Setting reminders or alarms can help you stay on track and ensure that you don't forget to follow through with your healthy habits.

Another strategy is to plan ahead and prepare for potential obstacles or challenges that may arise. This could involve meal prepping for the week, packing gym clothes the night before, or setting aside time for grocery shopping and meal planning.

It's also important to be flexible and willing to adjust your routine as needed. Life can be unpredictable, and unexpected events may disrupt your schedule from time to time. Instead of giving up when things don't go as planned, find alternative ways to incorporate your healthy habits into your day.

By creating a routine that prioritizes healthy behaviors and integrating them into your daily life, you can establish sustainable habits that contribute to your overall health and well-being. Over time, these habits will become second nature, making it easier to maintain a healthy lifestyle in the long run.

4. Monitor Your Progress:

Keep track of your actions and progress towards your goals. This can be done through journaling, using habit-tracking apps, or simply marking off each day on a calendar. Seeing your progress can provide motivation and reinforce your commitment to the habit.

Monitoring your progress is a vital strategy for building healthy habits as it provides valuable feedback, keeps you accountable, and helps you stay motivated towards your goals. There are several effective ways to monitor your progress and track your habits.

One approach is to keep a journal or log where you record your daily activities, including your healthy habits. This could involve writing down what you eat, how much exercise you do, or any other relevant behaviors you're trying to change. Reviewing your journal regularly allows you to track your progress over time and identify patterns or areas for improvement.

Another strategy is to use technology, such as habit-tracking apps or wearable fitness devices, to monitor your habits and progress automatically. These tools can provide real-time feedback, reminders, and insights into your behavior, making it easier to stay on track and make adjustments as needed.

Setting specific goals and milestones can also help you monitor your progress more effectively. By breaking down your larger goals into smaller, measurable objectives, you can track your progress more accurately and celebrate your achievements along the way.

Regularly reviewing your progress and reflecting on your successes and challenges can help you stay motivated and committed to your healthy habits. It's essential to celebrate your wins and acknowledge your efforts, even if progress is slow or incremental.

Overall, monitoring your progress is a powerful tool for building healthy habits and achieving your goals. By tracking your behaviors, staying accountable, and making adjustments as needed, you can create lasting changes that contribute to your overall health and well-being.

5. Stay Accountable:

Share your goals and progress with a friend, family member, or support group. Having someone to hold you accountable can help keep you motivated and accountable. You can also join online communities or forums related to your habit for additional support and encouragement.

Staying accountable is a crucial strategy for building healthy habits as it provides support, motivation, and encouragement to help you stay on track towards your goals. There are several effective ways to stay accountable in your journey towards developing healthy habits.

One approach is to find an accountability partner or buddy who shares similar goals and aspirations. This could be a friend, family member, or colleague who can offer support, guidance, and encouragement along the way. Regular check-ins, sharing progress updates, and celebrating successes together can help keep you motivated and accountable.

Joining a support group or community focused on health and wellness can also provide accountability and motivation. Whether it's an online forum, a local meet-up group, or a fitness class, being part of a community of like-minded individuals can offer encouragement, inspiration, and accountability.

Setting public commitments or declarations can help increase accountability by making your goals more visible and tangible. This could involve sharing your goals on social media, posting them in a prominent place at home or work, or publicly announcing your intentions to friends and family.

Using technology, such as habit-tracking apps or online accountability platforms, can also help you stay on track with your goals. These tools can provide reminders, progress tracking, and support from virtual communities, making it easier to stay accountable and motivated.

Overall, staying accountable is essential for building healthy habits and achieving your goals. By finding support, setting public commitments, and using technology to track your progress, you can stay motivated, focused, and committed to making positive changes in your life.

6. Reward Yourself:

Celebrate your successes along the way. Treat yourself to a small reward when you reach milestones or accomplish your goals. Positive reinforcement can help reinforce the habit and make it more enjoyable.

Rewarding yourself is a powerful strategy for building healthy habits as it provides positive reinforcement, motivation, and a sense of accomplishment. By incorporating rewards into your habit-building process, you can create a positive association with your new behaviors and increase your likelihood of sticking to them.

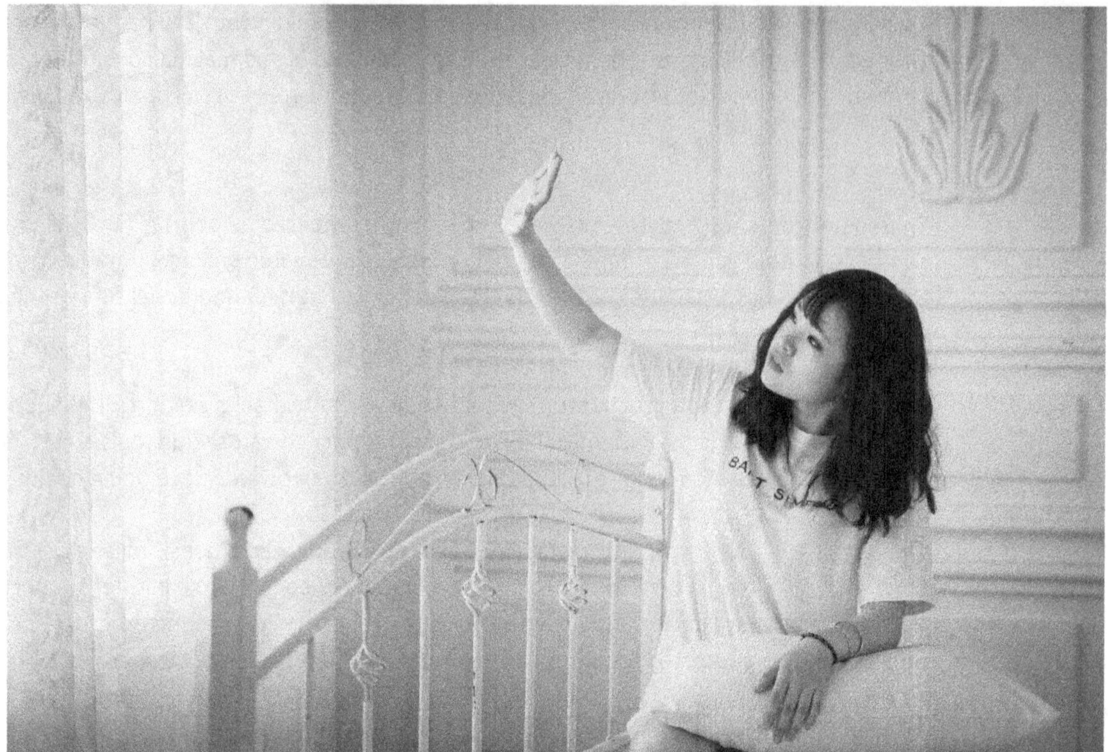

One approach is to set up a reward system where you designate specific rewards for achieving milestones or making progress towards your goals. These rewards can be anything that you find enjoyable or motivating, such as treating yourself to a massage, buying yourself a new outfit, or indulging in your favorite healthy snack.

It's essential to make sure that your rewards are aligned with your goals and don't undermine your progress. For example, if your goal is to eat healthier, rewarding yourself with a sugary dessert may not be the best choice. Instead, opt for rewards that support your overall well-being and reinforce your healthy habits.

In addition to larger rewards for reaching significant milestones, incorporating smaller, more frequent rewards for daily or weekly progress can help keep you motivated and engaged. This could involve giving yourself a pat on the back, enjoying a relaxing bath, or taking a break to do something you enjoy.

Overall, rewarding yourself for building healthy habits can make the process more enjoyable, sustainable, and rewarding. By celebrating your successes and acknowledging your efforts along the way, you can stay motivated and committed to making positive changes in your life.

7. Be Patient and Flexible:

Building healthy habits takes time and persistence. Be patient with yourself and don't get discouraged by setbacks. If you encounter obstacles or setbacks, adjust your approach and keep moving forward.

Being patient and flexible is a crucial strategy for building healthy habits as it allows for realistic expectations, resilience, and adaptability throughout the process of habit formation.

Developing new habits takes time, and it's important to recognize that progress may not happen overnight.

Practicing patience involves understanding that change is a gradual process and being kind to yourself during setbacks or periods of slow progress. It's essential to avoid becoming discouraged by temporary setbacks and to focus on the long-term benefits of your efforts.

Flexibility is also key when building healthy habits as it allows you to adjust your approach based on changing circumstances or feedback. If a particular strategy isn't working or if life gets in the way, being flexible enables you to adapt your plans and find alternative solutions.

Instead of viewing setbacks or deviations from your plan as failures, see them as opportunities for learning and growth. Reflect on what went wrong, identify potential barriers, and brainstorm alternative strategies to overcome them in the future.

By practicing patience and flexibility, you can navigate the ups and downs of habit formation with resilience and determination. Remember that building healthy habits is a journey, and it's okay to take small steps or make adjustments along the way.

Ultimately, cultivating patience and flexibility will help you stay motivated and committed to achieving your goals for long-term health and well-being.

8. Practice Self-compassion:

Be kind to yourself throughout the process. Acknowledge that change is hard, and it's okay to slip up occasionally. Instead of dwelling on failures, focus on what you've learned and how you can improve moving forward.

Practicing self-compassion is a crucial strategy for building healthy habits as it fosters kindness, understanding, and acceptance towards oneself throughout the habit-building process.

Developing new habits can be challenging, and it's essential to treat yourself with the same kindness and understanding that you would offer to a friend facing similar challenges.

Self-compassion involves recognizing that setbacks and struggles are a natural part of the journey towards building healthier habits. Instead of being overly critical or judgmental of yourself when things don't go as planned, practice self-compassion by offering yourself words of encouragement and support.

Be gentle with yourself during times of difficulty or temptation, and remember that perfection is not the goal. Acknowledge your efforts and progress, no matter how small, and celebrate your successes along the way.

Self-compassion also involves being mindful of your inner dialogue and challenging negative self-talk. Instead of dwelling on past mistakes or perceived failures, focus on learning from them and moving forward with a sense of self-acceptance and resilience.

By practicing self-compassion, you can cultivate a positive and nurturing relationship with yourself that supports your efforts to build healthier habits. Treat yourself with the same

kindness and understanding that you would offer to a loved one, and remember that you are worthy of compassion and support throughout your journey towards better health and well-being.

By incorporating these strategies into your daily life, you can gradually build and maintain healthy habits that contribute to your overall health and well-being. Remember that consistency and persistence are key, and small steps can lead to significant long-term changes.

5.3 Overcoming Obstacles and Staying Consistent

Overcoming obstacles and staying consistent are essential elements in the journey of building healthy habits. Challenges and setbacks are inevitable, but with the right strategies, individuals can navigate through them and maintain their commitment to their goals.

One effective approach to overcoming obstacles is to anticipate and plan for potential challenges in advance. This involves identifying common barriers that may arise, such as lack of time, stress, or temptation, and brainstorming strategies to address them.

For example, if time constraints are a barrier to exercising regularly, scheduling workouts at a specific time each day or breaking them into shorter sessions can help overcome this obstacle.

Another strategy is to cultivate resilience and a growth mindset. Instead of viewing setbacks as failures, see them as opportunities for learning and growth.

Reflect on what went wrong, identify factors that contributed to the setback, and adjust your approach accordingly. Remember that progress is not always linear, and setbacks are a natural part of the process.

Seeking support from others can also help overcome obstacles and stay consistent. Whether it's enlisting the help of a friend, family member, or coach, having someone to provide encouragement, accountability, and perspective can make a significant difference.

 Additionally, joining a support group or community of like-minded individuals can offer valuable insights, motivation, and inspiration to overcome challenges and stay on track.

To stay consistent, it's essential to establish routines and habits that align with your goals. Consistency is key to building healthy habits, as it helps reinforce behaviors and make them automatic. Set specific goals, create a plan of action, and commit to sticking to it, even when faced with obstacles or temptations.

Finally, practice self-compassion and patience throughout the process. Be kind to yourself during setbacks, and acknowledge your efforts and progress, no matter how small. Remember that building healthy habits is a journey, and it's okay to take one step at a time.

By overcoming obstacles and staying consistent, individuals can achieve their goals and experience lasting changes in their health and well-being.

Chapter 6: Sleep and Stress Management

Sleep and stress management are two critical components of maintaining overall health and well-being. Both play significant roles in various aspects of physical, mental, and emotional health, and addressing them effectively can lead to improved quality of life.

Sleep is essential for the body's ability to function optimally. It plays a vital role in processes such as memory consolidation, immune function, hormone regulation, and mood regulation. Insufficient or poor-quality sleep can lead to a range of health issues, including impaired cognitive function, increased risk of chronic diseases such as obesity and diabetes, and heightened stress levels.

To improve sleep quality and duration, individuals can implement several strategies. Establishing a consistent sleep schedule, where bedtime and wake-up times are the same each day, helps regulate the body's internal clock and promote better sleep patterns.

Creating a relaxing bedtime routine, such as reading a book, taking a warm bath, or practicing relaxation techniques like deep breathing or meditation, can signal to the body that it's time to wind down and prepare for sleep. Additionally, creating a comfortable sleep environment, free from distractions such as noise and light, can further enhance sleep quality.

Effective stress management is also crucial for overall well-being. Chronic stress can have detrimental effects on both physical and mental health, contributing to issues such as high blood pressure,

weakened immune function, anxiety, and depression. Learning to manage stress effectively is essential for mitigating these negative effects and promoting resilience in the face of life's challenges.

Several strategies can help individuals manage stress more effectively. Regular physical activity, such as exercise or yoga, can help reduce stress hormones and promote feelings of relaxation and well-being.

Practicing mindfulness and meditation can help individuals cultivate present-moment awareness and develop coping skills for managing stressors. Additionally, maintaining a healthy lifestyle, including balanced nutrition, adequate hydration, and regular relaxation techniques, can support the body's ability to cope with stress more effectively.

In summary, prioritizing sleep and stress management is essential for maintaining overall health and well-being. By implementing strategies to improve sleep quality and duration and effectively managing stress, individuals can enhance their physical, mental, and emotional resilience and enjoy a higher quality of life.

5.1 Importance of Sleep for Weight Loss

Sleep plays a crucial role in weight loss and overall metabolic health. Several mechanisms contribute to this relationship, highlighting the importance of adequate sleep for successful weight management.

Firstly, sleep deprivation can disrupt hormonal balance, leading to increased levels of hunger hormones such as ghrelin and decreased levels of satiety hormones like leptin. This imbalance can result in heightened appetite, cravings for high-calorie foods, and ultimately, overeating, which can hinder weight loss efforts.

Moreover, inadequate sleep can impair glucose metabolism and insulin sensitivity, increasing the risk of insulin resistance and type 2 diabetes. This can lead to elevated blood sugar levels and greater storage of fat, particularly around the abdominal area, further complicating weight loss goals.

Additionally, sleep deprivation can negatively impact energy levels, motivation, and cognitive function, making it more challenging to engage in physical activity and make healthy food choices. Reduced exercise and poor dietary decisions can impede weight loss progress and undermine efforts to achieve a calorie deficit.

Overall, prioritizing sufficient sleep is essential for supporting optimal hormonal balance, metabolic function, and energy levels, all of which are critical for successful weight loss. By ensuring adequate rest and quality sleep, individuals can enhance their ability to make healthy lifestyle choices, manage appetite and cravings, and achieve their weight loss goals more effectively.

5.2 Strategies for Improving Sleep Quality

Improving sleep quality involves adopting various strategies to create an environment and routine conducive to restful and rejuvenating sleep. Here are some effective strategies:

1. Establish a Consistent Sleep Schedule:
   Going to bed and waking up at the same time every day, even on weekends, helps regulate your body's internal clock and promote a consistent sleep-wake cycle.

   Establishing a consistent sleep schedule involves going to bed and waking up at the same time every day, including weekends. This routine helps regulate your body's internal clock, known as the circadian rhythm, promoting better sleep quality and overall health.

   Consistency reinforces your body's natural sleep-wake cycle, making it easier to fall asleep and wake up refreshed. Over time, sticking to a consistent sleep schedule can improve sleep efficiency,

   enhance daytime alertness, and reduce the risk of sleep disorders. It's an essential strategy for maintaining optimal sleep patterns and promoting overall well-being.

2. Create a Relaxing Bedtime Routine:
   Engage in relaxing activities before bedtime to signal to your body that it's time to wind down. This could include reading a book, taking a warm bath, practicing meditation or deep breathing exercises, or listening to calming music.

   Creating a relaxing bedtime routine involves engaging in calming activities before sleep to signal to your body that it's time to wind down. This routine can include activities such as reading a book, taking a warm bath, practicing gentle stretching or yoga, or listening to soothing music.

By incorporating these relaxing activities into your nightly routine, you can help quiet your mind, reduce stress and anxiety, and prepare your body for restful sleep.

Consistently practicing a bedtime routine can promote better sleep quality and help you unwind after a busy day, leading to improved overall well-being.

3. Create a Comfortable Sleep Environment:
    Ensure that your bedroom is conducive to sleep by keeping it dark, quiet, and cool. Invest in a comfortable mattress and pillows, and consider using blackout curtains, white noise machines, or earplugs to minimize disturbances.

    Creating a comfortable sleep environment involves optimizing your bedroom to promote restful and uninterrupted sleep. Start by ensuring your mattress and pillows provide adequate support and comfort.

    Use soft, breathable bedding and maintain a comfortable room temperature, typically between 60-67°F (15-20°C).

    Minimize noise and light disturbances by using blackout curtains or a white noise machine. Keep electronics out of the bedroom and consider dimming the lights before bedtime to signal to your body that it's time to sleep.

    By creating a peaceful and comfortable sleep environment, you can enhance sleep quality and wake up feeling refreshed and rejuvenated each morning.

4. Limit Screen Time Before Bed:
    The blue light emitted by screens can interfere with your body's production of melatonin, a hormone that regulates sleep. Try to avoid electronic devices such as smartphones, tablets, and computers at least an hour before bedtime.

    Limiting screen time before bed is crucial for improving sleep quality. The blue light emitted by screens, such as smartphones, tablets, and computers, can disrupt the production of melatonin,

    a hormone that regulates sleep-wake cycles. Engaging with screens close to bedtime can delay the onset of sleep and reduce overall sleep duration.

    To promote better sleep, establish a "screen curfew" by avoiding electronic devices at least an hour before bed. Instead, opt for relaxing activities such as reading a book or practicing relaxation techniques. By minimizing screen time before bed, you can improve sleep quality and overall well-being.

5. Watch Your Diet and Hydration:
   Avoid heavy meals, caffeine, and alcohol close to bedtime, as they can disrupt sleep patterns. Instead, opt for light snacks and herbal teas that promote relaxation and hydration.

   Watching your diet and hydration is essential for promoting quality sleep. Avoid heavy meals, caffeine, and alcohol close to bedtime, as they can disrupt sleep patterns and cause discomfort. Instead, opt for light snacks and herbal teas that promote relaxation and hydration.

   Maintaining proper hydration throughout the day can prevent night time awakenings due to thirst. Additionally, consuming a balanced diet rich in whole foods, fruits,

   and vegetables supports overall health and can contribute to better sleep quality. By being mindful of your diet and hydration habits, you can create optimal conditions for restful and rejuvenating sleep.

6. Manage Stress and Anxiety:
   Practice stress-reducing techniques such as mindfulness, meditation, or progressive muscle relaxation to calm your mind and prepare for sleep.

   Managing stress and anxiety is crucial for promoting quality sleep. High levels of stress and anxiety can lead to difficulty falling asleep, staying asleep, and experiencing restorative sleep.

   To manage stress, practice relaxation techniques such as deep breathing, meditation, or progressive muscle relaxation. Engage in regular physical activity,

   which can help reduce stress hormones and promote relaxation. Additionally, establish healthy coping mechanisms such as journaling, talking to a trusted friend or therapist, or engaging in enjoyable activities.

   By effectively managing stress and anxiety, you can create a calmer mind and body, leading to improved sleep quality and overall well-being.

By incorporating these strategies into your daily routine, you can create a conducive environment for restful and rejuvenating sleep, leading to improved sleep quality and overall well-being.

Managing Stress for Weight Management

Managing stress is essential for effective weight management as chronic stress can significantly impact eating behaviors, metabolism, and overall health. When stress levels are high, the body releases cortisol, a hormone that can lead to increased appetite and cravings for high-calorie, sugary foods. These behaviors can contribute to weight gain and difficulty in losing weight.

To manage stress effectively for weight management, it's important to adopt various strategies that address both the physical and psychological aspects of stress.

One approach is to incorporate regular physical activity into your routine. Exercise has been shown to reduce stress hormones like cortisol and release endorphins, which are natural mood elevators.

Engaging in activities such as walking, yoga, or strength training can help alleviate stress and promote overall well-being.

Additionally, practicing relaxation techniques such as deep breathing, meditation, or progressive muscle relaxation can help reduce stress levels and promote relaxation. These techniques can be particularly beneficial when practiced regularly as part of a daily routine.

Maintaining a healthy lifestyle, including balanced nutrition and adequate sleep, is also crucial for managing stress and supporting weight management efforts.

Eating a balanced diet rich in fruits, vegetables, whole grains, and lean proteins can provide essential nutrients that support the body's ability to cope with stress. Adequate sleep is also important, as poor sleep quality can exacerbate stress levels and impact weight management.

Furthermore, it's essential to develop healthy coping mechanisms for dealing with stressors. This may involve setting boundaries, practicing assertiveness, seeking social support, or seeking professional help from a therapist or counselor.

Learning to manage stress effectively can help prevent emotional eating and other unhealthy coping behaviors that can sabotage weight management efforts.

In summary, managing stress is crucial for effective weight management. By incorporating regular physical activity, practicing relaxation techniques, maintaining a healthy lifestyle,

and developing healthy coping mechanisms, individuals can reduce stress levels, support overall well-being, and achieve their weight management goals more effectively.

Chapter 7: Tracking Progress

Tracking progress is an essential component of any goal-setting and achievement process, providing valuable insights into one's journey and motivating further improvement. Whether it's in weight loss, fitness, career development, or personal growth, monitoring progress allows individuals to stay accountable, identify areas for improvement, and celebrate successes along the way.

One of the primary benefits of tracking progress is that it provides tangible evidence of growth and improvement over time. By regularly recording data, such as weight, measurements, or performance metrics, individuals can see how far they've come and stay motivated to continue their efforts.

Tracking progress also helps individuals identify patterns and trends that may impact their success. By analyzing data over time, individuals can gain valuable insights into what strategies are working well and where adjustments may be needed.

For example, someone trying to lose weight may notice that their progress stalls when they eat out frequently, prompting them to focus on meal planning and preparation at home.

Additionally, tracking progress allows individuals to set realistic goals and benchmarks based on their current performance. By setting specific, measurable targets, individuals can track their progress more effectively and make adjustments as needed to stay on track towards their ultimate goals.

Moreover, tracking progress provides accountability and helps individuals stay committed to their goals. Knowing that they have to record their progress regularly can motivate individuals to stay consistent with their efforts and make healthier choices.

There are various methods for tracking progress, including journaling, using apps or online tools, or keeping a visual progress chart. The key is to choose a method that works best for you and allows you to track relevant metrics easily and accurately.

In summary, tracking progress is a powerful tool for achieving success in any endeavor. By regularly monitoring and recording data, individuals can stay motivated, identify areas for improvement, and make informed decisions to reach their goals more effectively. Whether it's in health and fitness, career development, or personal growth, tracking progress is an essential strategy for success.

6.1 Tracking Food Intake

Tracking food intake is a valuable strategy for promoting healthy eating habits, managing weight, and achieving nutritional goals. By keeping a record of the foods and beverages consumed throughout the day, individuals can gain insight into their dietary patterns, identify areas for improvement, and make informed decisions about their nutrition.

There are various methods for tracking food intake, ranging from traditional pen-and-paper journals to mobile apps and online tools. These tools allow individuals to log their meals, snacks, portion sizes, and even nutritional information such as calories, macronutrients, and micronutrients.

Tracking food intake helps individuals become more mindful of their eating habits, allowing them to recognize patterns such as emotional eating, mindless snacking, or consuming excessive portions. This awareness empowers individuals to make healthier choices and adopt more balanced and nutritious eating habits over time.

Moreover, tracking food intake can support weight management efforts by providing accountability and helping individuals stay within their calorie or macronutrient targets. By monitoring their food intake regularly, individuals can adjust their eating habits as needed to achieve their weight loss, maintenance, or muscle-building goals.

Overall, tracking food intake is a powerful tool for promoting healthy eating habits and achieving nutritional goals. Whether it's for weight management, improving overall health, or addressing specific dietary concerns, keeping track of food intake can provide valuable insights and support long-term success in maintaining a balanced and nutritious diet.

7.2 Monitoring Physical Activity

Monitoring physical activity is essential for maintaining an active lifestyle, achieving fitness goals, and promoting overall health and well-being. By keeping track of their activity levels, individuals can assess their progress, identify areas for improvement, and stay motivated to engage in regular exercise.

There are various methods for monitoring physical activity, ranging from simple pen-and-paper logs to sophisticated wearable devices and fitness apps. These tools allow individuals to track metrics such as steps taken, distance traveled, duration of exercise sessions, and calories burned.

Monitoring physical activity provides individuals with valuable feedback on their exercise habits, allowing them to identify patterns and trends in their activity levels. This insight can help individuals set realistic goals, track their progress over time, and make adjustments to their exercise routine as needed.

Additionally, monitoring physical activity can help individuals stay accountable and motivated to stick to their fitness regimen. By seeing their activity levels and progress displayed visually, individuals can stay focused on their goals and celebrate their achievements along the way.

Moreover, monitoring physical activity allows individuals to track their adherence to recommended guidelines for physical activity and exercise. This can help ensure that individuals are meeting their daily or weekly targets for aerobic exercise, strength training, and overall physical activity, leading to improved fitness and health outcomes.

Overall, monitoring physical activity is a valuable tool for promoting an active lifestyle, achieving fitness goals, and maintaining overall health and well-being. Whether it's through simple tracking methods or advanced wearable technology, monitoring physical activity allows individuals to stay engaged, motivated, and accountable to their exercise routine.

7.3 Celebrating Non-Scale Victories

Celebrating non-scale victories is a powerful practice that focuses on recognizing and acknowledging progress and achievements in areas beyond just the number on the scale. While weight loss is often a primary goal for many individuals, non-scale victories encompass a broader range of accomplishments related to health, fitness, and overall well-being.

These victories can include improvements in energy levels, increased strength and endurance, better sleep quality, enhanced mood and mental clarity, clothing fitting better, and achieving personal fitness milestones such as running a certain distance or lifting heavier weights. Additionally, non-scale victories may involve positive changes in habits and behaviors, such as making healthier food choices, sticking to an exercise routine, or practicing self-care and stress management techniques.

Celebrating non-scale victories is important because it reinforces progress and boosts motivation, regardless of fluctuations in weight. It shifts the focus from solely relying on the scale as a measure of success to recognizing the many other positive

changes occurring as a result of adopting healthier habits. By celebrating these victories, individuals cultivate a more positive mindset, build confidence, and feel empowered to continue their journey towards improved health and well-being.

Chapter 8: Overcoming Plateaus and Setbacks

Overcoming plateaus and setbacks is an inevitable part of any journey towards achieving goals, including weight loss, fitness, or personal development. Plateaus occur when progress stalls or slows down, while setbacks involve temporary regressions or obstacles that hinder forward movement. Here are some strategies for overcoming plateaus and setbacks:

Overcoming plateaus and setbacks is an integral part of any journey towards personal growth and success. Plateaus, where progress seems to stall despite continued efforts, can be frustrating, but they also present opportunities for reflection and adjustment. One effective strategy is to reassess goals and methods, seeking out new approaches or techniques to break through the plateau.

Setbacks, whether they're minor obstacles or major challenges, are inevitable in any endeavor. The key to overcoming them lies in resilience and adaptability. Instead of dwelling on setbacks, it's important to view them as learning experiences and opportunities for growth. Analyzing what went wrong, identifying lessons learned, and devising a plan to move forward can help turn setbacks into stepping stones towards eventual success.

Moreover, maintaining a positive mindset and seeking support from others can bolster your resilience during challenging times. By embracing setbacks as temporary setbacks rather than permanent failures, you can harness their transformative power to propel yourself forward on your journey.

1. Assess and Adjust:

    Take a step back to evaluate your current strategies and identify potential reasons for the plateau or setback. Reflect on factors such as changes in routine, stress levels, nutrition, and exercise habits.

    Based on your assessment, make adjustments to your approach, such as modifying your workout routine, reassessing your dietary choices, or seeking support from a mentor or coach.

    Assessing and adjusting is a crucial strategy for overcoming plateaus and setbacks in various aspects of life, including fitness, weight loss, career, or personal development.

    This strategy involves taking a step back to evaluate your current situation objectively and making necessary adjustments to your approach to keep moving forward towards your goals.

    To begin, assess your progress and identify any factors that may be contributing to the plateau or setback. This could include changes in routine, lack of consistency, external stressors, or ineffective strategies. Be honest with yourself and gather data to gain a clear understanding of what's working and what's not.

    Once you've identified areas for improvement, make adjustments to your approach accordingly. This could involve modifying your workout routine, reassessing your dietary choices,

    seeking additional support or guidance, or changing your mindset and perspective. Keep an open mind and be willing to try new strategies or approaches to overcome obstacles and break through plateaus.

Regularly reassessing and adjusting your approach is essential for staying adaptable and responsive to changing circumstances. By being proactive and flexible in your approach, you can overcome plateaus and setbacks more effectively and continue making progress towards your goals.

Remember that progress is not always linear, and setbacks are a natural part of the journey towards growth and improvement. Stay patient, persistent, and committed to your goals, and be willing to adjust your course as needed to achieve success.

2. Set Realistic Expectations:

Recognize that plateaus and setbacks are normal and to be expected on any journey towards improvement. Instead of becoming discouraged, view them as opportunities for growth and learning. Adjust your expectations and focus on progress rather than perfection, celebrating small victories along the way.

Setting realistic expectations is vital for navigating through plateaus and setbacks effectively. It involves acknowledging the possibility of challenges and setbacks along the journey toward achieving goals and understanding that progress may not always be linear.

To set realistic expectations, it's essential to assess your starting point, resources, and capabilities realistically. Consider factors such as your current fitness level, available time, and potential obstacles you may encounter along the way. Set goals that are challenging yet achievable, taking into account your personal circumstances and limitations.

Additionally, recognize that progress takes time and that setbacks are a normal part of any transformative process. Rather than expecting immediate results, focus on making

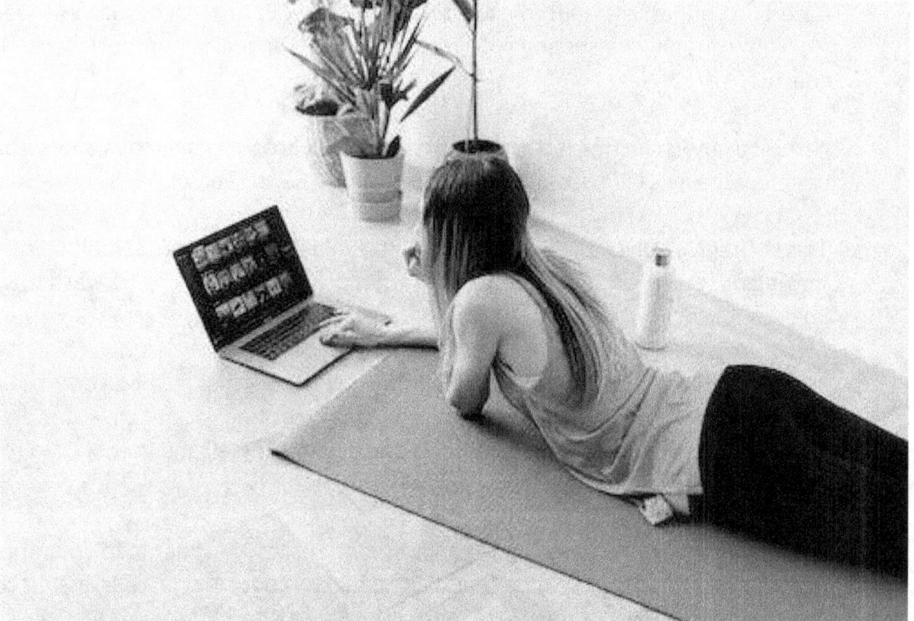

incremental progress and celebrating small victories along the way. This approach can help you stay motivated and maintain momentum, even when faced with challenges or setbacks.

Moreover, it's crucial to cultivate a growth mindset and view setbacks as opportunities for learning and growth rather than failures. Embrace the journey and be willing to adapt your approach as needed to overcome obstacles and continue making progress toward your goals.

By setting realistic expectations, acknowledging the possibility of setbacks, and adopting a growth mindset, you can navigate through plateaus and setbacks with resilience and determination, ultimately achieving success in your endeavors.

3. Stay Consistent:

Consistency is key to overcoming plateaus and setbacks. Stick to your routine, even when progress seems slow or non-existent. Trust the process and remain committed to your goals, knowing that consistent effort over time will yield results.

Staying consistent is a key factor in overcoming plateaus and setbacks effectively. Consistency involves maintaining a steady effort and dedication to your goals, even when faced with challenges or setbacks along the way.

Consistency is essential because it allows you to build momentum and progress steadily towards your objectives. By committing to regular practice, whether it's exercising, studying, or working towards a goal, you create habits that reinforce positive behaviors and contribute to long-term success.

Moreover, consistency helps you overcome plateaus by pushing through periods of stagnation and maintaining forward momentum. Even when progress seems slow or non-existent, staying consistent with your efforts ensures that you continue moving in the right direction.

Consistency also builds discipline and resilience, enabling you to persevere through obstacles and setbacks with determination. It fosters a mindset of commitment and dedication, where you prioritize your goals and stay focused on achieving them, regardless of challenges or distractions that may arise.

Additionally, staying consistent helps you develop trust in yourself and your abilities. When you consistently show up and put in the work, you build confidence in your capacity to overcome obstacles and achieve success, fueling further motivation and perseverance.

In summary, staying consistent is essential for overcoming plateaus and setbacks because it builds momentum, maintains progress, fosters discipline and resilience, and cultivates trust in oneself.

By staying committed to your goals and maintaining consistent effort, you can navigate through challenges and setbacks with determination and ultimately achieve success in your endeavors.

4. Mix Things Up:

Plateaus often occur when the body adapts to a certain routine or stimulus. Shake things up by trying new exercises, varying your intensity or duration, or exploring different workout modalities. This can help challenge your body in new ways and break through plateaus.

Mixing things up is a valuable strategy for overcoming plateaus and setbacks in various areas of life, including fitness, personal development, and professional growth. When progress stagnates or obstacles arise, introducing variety and change into your routine can help break through barriers and reignite motivation.

One way to mix things up is by trying new activities or exercises that challenge your body in different ways. This could involve incorporating new workout routines, exploring different fitness classes,

or engaging in alternative forms of exercise such as swimming, cycling, or yoga. Changing up your routine can stimulate new muscle groups, prevent boredom, and overcome plateaus in fitness progress.

Additionally, mixing things up can involve adjusting your approach or mindset towards your goals. Instead of sticking to the same strategies that may not be yielding results, be open to experimenting with different techniques or perspectives.

This could mean seeking advice from mentors or experts, trying out new problem-solving methods, or exploring alternative paths towards your objectives.

Furthermore, mixing things up can extend beyond physical activities to include changes in your environment, social interactions, or daily habits. Incorporating new experiences, hobbies, or social activities can provide a refreshing break from routine and spark creativity and inspiration.

By mixing things up and embracing change, you can overcome plateaus and setbacks more effectively, keep motivation levels high, and continue progressing towards your goals with renewed energy and enthusiasm.

5. Practice Patience and Persistence:
Overcoming plateaus and setbacks requires patience and persistence. Stay focused on your long-term goals and keep moving forward, even when progress seems slow. Remember that setbacks are temporary, and with perseverance, you can overcome them and continue making progress towards your goals.

Practicing patience and persistence is essential when facing plateaus and setbacks in any endeavor. It involves maintaining a steadfast commitment to your goals and understanding that progress may not always happen as quickly or smoothly as desired.

Patience is the ability to tolerate delays, obstacles, and difficulties without becoming frustrated or discouraged. It allows you to maintain a long-term perspective, recognizing that meaningful change takes time and perseverance.

Instead of expecting immediate results, practicing patience involves trusting the process and remaining focused on your goals, even when faced with challenges or setbacks.

Persistence is the determination to continue moving forward despite obstacles or setbacks. It involves resilience in the face of adversity, refusing to give up in the face of challenges, and staying committed to your objectives.

Rather than being deterred by setbacks, persistent individuals view them as opportunities for growth and learning, using setbacks as motivation to keep pushing forward.

Together, patience and persistence form a powerful mindset that enables individuals to navigate through plateaus and setbacks with resilience and determination. By practicing patience, you can maintain a sense of calm and perspective during challenging times,

while persistence empowers you to keep taking action and moving towards your goals, even when progress seems slow or difficult. Ultimately, cultivating these qualities can lead to greater success and fulfillment in achieving your objectives.

Seek Support:

Don't hesitate to reach out for support from friends, family, or a professional if you're feeling stuck or discouraged. Surround yourself with a supportive network of individuals who can offer encouragement, advice, and accountability to help you overcome plateaus and setbacks.

Seeking support is a valuable strategy for overcoming plateaus and setbacks in various aspects of life, including personal goals, career aspirations, and health and wellness endeavors. When facing challenges or obstacles, reaching out for help can provide valuable guidance, encouragement, and perspective to help navigate through difficult times.

can come in many forms, including seeking advice from mentors, coaches, or experts in your field. These individuals can offer insights, strategies, and encouragement based on their own experiences and expertise, helping you overcome obstacles and make progress towards your goals more effectively.

Additionally, seeking support from friends, family members, or peers can provide emotional encouragement and motivation during challenging times. Simply talking about your struggles and receiving validation and empathy from others can help alleviate feelings of isolation and boost morale.

Furthermore, joining a support group or community of like-minded individuals can offer a sense of camaraderie and shared experiences. Connecting with others who are facing similar challenges can provide encouragement, accountability, and inspiration to keep moving forward, even when faced with setbacks or difficulties.

By seeking support from others, you can gain valuable insights, encouragement, and motivation to overcome plateaus and setbacks, ultimately helping you achieve success in your endeavors. Remember that it's okay to ask for help and lean on others for support when needed, as we are all stronger together.

By implementing these strategies, you can overcome plateaus and setbacks, stay motivated, and continue making progress towards your goals, ultimately achieving success in your journey of self-improvement.

8.1 Understanding Weight Loss Plateaus

Weight loss plateaus are common occurrences during the process of losing weight, characterized by a temporary stall or slowdown in weight loss progress despite continued efforts. Understanding the factors contributing to these plateaus can help individuals navigate through them more effectively.

One factor contributing to weight loss plateaus is metabolic adaptation, where the body adjusts to a lower calorie intake by reducing metabolic rate. This can occur as a result of prolonged calorie restriction or significant weight loss, making it harder to continue losing weight at the same rate.

Additionally, changes in hormone levels, such as leptin and ghrelin, can influence hunger and satiety signals, potentially leading to increased appetite and reduced energy expenditure. This can contribute to overeating and hinder weight loss progress.

Furthermore, factors such as stress, lack of sleep, and changes in activity levels can impact weight loss efforts. Stress hormones like cortisol can promote fat storage and cravings for high-calorie foods, while inadequate sleep can disrupt metabolic function and increase hunger levels.

To overcome weight loss plateaus, individuals can try adjusting their calorie intake, increasing physical activity levels, or incorporating more variety into their diet and exercise routine.

Additionally, focusing on non-scale victories, such as improvements in energy levels, strength, and overall well-being, can help maintain motivation and momentum during plateaus. Understanding that weight loss is not always linear and being patient and persistent in efforts to achieve long-term success is key.

Breaking through plateaus requires a strategic approach that involves reassessing your current methods, making adjustments, and persisting in your efforts. Here are some effective strategies for overcoming plateaus in various areas of life:

1. Adjust Your Routine:

    Introduce changes to your workout routine by incorporating new exercises, increasing intensity, or varying your workout schedule. This can shock your body out of its plateau and stimulate new muscle growth or fat loss.

    Adjusting your routine is a key strategy for breaking through plateaus in various aspects of life, including fitness, career, and personal development. When progress stalls or slows down, making changes to your routine can help stimulate new growth, overcome obstacles, and reignite motivation.

    In the context of fitness, adjusting your routine involves introducing variations to your workouts to challenge your body in different ways. This could include trying new exercises,

    increasing the intensity or duration of your workouts, or changing your workout schedule. By constantly challenging your muscles with new stimuli, you can prevent adaptation and continue making progress towards your fitness goals.

    Similarly, in career or personal development pursuits, adjusting your routine may involve reevaluating your daily habits and making changes to optimize productivity and effectiveness. This could include prioritizing tasks differently, experimenting with new strategies or techniques, or seeking out additional learning opportunities.

The key to successfully adjusting your routine is to be flexible and open-minded, willing to experiment with different approaches to find what works best for you.

By embracing change and being proactive in making adjustments, you can break through plateaus, overcome obstacles, and continue moving forward towards your goals with renewed energy and momentum.

2. Focus on Nutrition:

Reevaluate your dietary habits and make adjustments to your calorie intake or macronutrient ratios. Incorporate more whole, nutrient-dense foods while reducing processed foods and empty calories.

Focusing on nutrition is essential for breaking through plateaus in weight loss, fitness, and overall health. Reevaluating your dietary habits and making adjustments can help overcome stagnant progress.

This involves prioritizing nutrient-dense foods, monitoring portion sizes, and balancing macronutrients to support your goals. Incorporating more whole foods, such as fruits, vegetables, lean proteins, and healthy fats, while minimizing processed foods and added sugars,

can optimize your nutrition and fuel your body for success. By paying attention to what you eat and making mindful choices, you can break through plateaus and achieve your desired outcomes.

3. Increase Intensity:

Push yourself to work harder during workouts by increasing the intensity or duration of your exercises. This can help rev up your metabolism and break through fitness plateaus.

Increasing intensity is a powerful strategy for breaking through plateaus in fitness and performance. By pushing yourself to work harder during workouts, you can challenge your muscles and cardiovascular system, leading to greater gains in strength, endurance, and overall fitness.

This can involve lifting heavier weights, performing more reps or sets, increasing resistance or speed, or reducing rest periods between exercises.

By progressively overloading your body with higher levels of intensity, you can stimulate further adaptation and growth, breaking through plateaus and reaching new levels of performance and physical fitness.

4. **Rest and Recovery:**

Ensure you're allowing your body enough time to rest and recover between workouts. Incorporate rest days into your routine and prioritize quality sleep to support muscle repair and overall recovery.

Rest and recovery are essential components of any successful training program, especially when aiming to break through plateaus in fitness. Allowing your body enough time to rest and recuperate between workouts is crucial for optimal muscle repair, growth, and overall recovery.

This involves incorporating rest days into your routine and prioritizing quality sleep to support physiological processes that occur during rest. Additionally, practicing relaxation techniques such as stretching,

foam rolling, or meditation can further enhance recovery and reduce the risk of overtraining. By prioritizing rest and recovery, you can ensure your body is adequately prepared to perform at its best and break through plateaus effectively.

5. **Set New Goals:**

Shift your focus to different goals or milestones to keep yourself motivated and engaged. This could involve aiming for a new personal best in a fitness-related activity or setting non-scale goals related to improved performance or well-being.

Setting new goals is a powerful strategy for breaking through plateaus and reinvigorating motivation. When faced with stagnant progress, shifting your focus to different objectives can provide a fresh sense of purpose and direction.

This could involve setting specific, measurable, achievable, relevant, and time-bound (SMART) goals related to different aspects of your journey, such as fitness, career, or personal development. By setting new challenges and milestones,

you can reignite enthusiasm and commitment, inspiring renewed effort and determination to overcome obstacles and achieve success. Embrace the opportunity to expand your horizons and push yourself to new heights by setting ambitious yet attainable goals.

6. **Seek Support:**

Reach out to friends, family, or professionals for encouragement, advice, and accountability. Surrounding yourself with a supportive network can provide the motivation and guidance needed to push through plateaus.

Seeking support is a vital strategy for breaking through plateaus and overcoming challenges in various areas of life. Whether pursuing fitness goals, career aspirations, or personal development endeavors, reaching out for assistance can provide valuable guidance, encouragement, and motivation.

Support can come in many forms, including seeking advice from mentors, coaches, or experts in your field. These individuals can offer insights, strategies, and accountability based on their own experiences and expertise, helping you navigate obstacles and make progress toward your goals more effectively.

Additionally, seeking support from friends, family members, or peers can provide emotional encouragement and motivation during difficult times. Simply sharing your struggles and receiving validation and empathy from others can help alleviate feelings of isolation and boost morale.

Furthermore, joining a support group or community of like-minded individuals can offer a sense of camaraderie and shared experiences. Connecting with others who are facing similar challenges can provide encouragement, accountability, and inspiration to keep moving forward, even when faced with setbacks or obstacles.

By seeking support from others, you can gain valuable insights, encouragement, and motivation to break through plateaus and achieve success in your endeavors. Remember that it's okay to ask for help and lean on others for support when needed, as we are all stronger together.

By implementing these strategies and staying persistent in your efforts, you can overcome plateaus and continue making progress towards your goals. Remember that plateaus are a natural part of any journey, and with patience, determination, and strategic adjustments, you can break through them and achieve success.

8.3 Dealing with Setbacks

Dealing with setbacks is an inevitable part of any journey towards achieving goals, whether in fitness, career, or personal development. Setbacks can be discouraging and challenging, but how you respond to them can significantly impact your ability to overcome obstacles and ultimately succeed.

Firstly, it's important to acknowledge and accept setbacks as a natural part of the process. Avoid dwelling on feelings of frustration or disappointment, and instead, view setbacks as opportunities for growth and learning. Recognize that setbacks are temporary and do not define your overall progress or potential for success.

Next, take a step back to evaluate the setback objectively. Identify the factors that contributed to the setback and consider what lessons can be learned from the experience. Reflect on any mistakes or areas for improvement, and use this information to adjust your approach and make informed decisions moving forward.

Maintaining a positive mindset is crucial when dealing with setbacks. Focus on the progress you've made so far and the lessons you've learned along the way. Remind yourself of your strengths, resilience, and ability to overcome challenges. By maintaining a positive outlook, you can stay motivated and resilient in the face of adversity.

Seeking support from others can also be instrumental in dealing with setbacks. Reach out to friends, family, mentors, or colleagues for encouragement, advice, and perspective. Sharing your struggles with others can provide emotional support and help you gain new insights into your situation.

Finally, take proactive steps to get back on track towards your goals. Set small, achievable goals to regain momentum and build confidence. Break down larger tasks into manageable steps and focus on making progress one day at a time. By taking action and staying committed to your goals, you can overcome setbacks and continue moving forward on your journey to success. Remember that setbacks are temporary roadblocks, not permanent barriers, and with resilience, perseverance, and determination, you can overcome them and achieve your goals.

Chapter 9: Building a Support System

Building a support system is a crucial aspect of personal growth and success in various areas of life. Whether pursuing fitness goals, career aspirations, or personal development endeavors, having a strong support system can provide encouragement, guidance, and motivation to help you navigate challenges and achieve your objectives.

One of the first steps in building a support system is identifying individuals who can offer meaningful support and guidance. This may include friends, family members, mentors, colleagues, or coaches who possess relevant expertise, experience, or insight into your goals and aspirations.

Once you've identified potential sources of support, it's important to cultivate and nurture these relationships. This involves communicating openly and honestly about your goals, aspirations, and challenges, and seeking input and advice from your support network when needed.

Additionally, reciprocity is key in building a support system. Offer your support and encouragement to others in your network, and be willing to listen, provide guidance, and offer assistance when they face challenges or setbacks. Building mutually supportive relationships creates a strong sense of community and fosters a supportive environment where everyone can thrive.

Furthermore, don't hesitate to seek out additional sources of support beyond your immediate circle. This may include joining online communities, forums, or support groups related to your goals or interests. Connecting with like-minded individuals who share similar aspirations can provide valuable encouragement, accountability, and camaraderie.

Finally, remember to express gratitude and appreciation for the support you receive from others. Recognize the contributions of your support system and show your appreciation through words of thanks, acts of kindness, or gestures of support. Building a culture of appreciation strengthens relationships and fosters a positive, supportive environment for personal growth and success.

In summary, building a support system is essential for achieving personal growth and success. By cultivating meaningful relationships, offering support to others, and seeking out additional sources of encouragement and guidance, you can create a strong support network that empowers you to overcome challenges, pursue your goals, and achieve your aspirations.

9.1 Importance of Social Support

Social support plays a crucial role in various aspects of life, including physical and mental health, personal development, and overall well-being. Having a strong support network provides numerous benefits that contribute to resilience, happiness, and success.

Firstly, social support offers emotional encouragement and validation during challenging times. Knowing that you have people who care about you and are there to listen and offer empathy can provide a sense of comfort and reassurance, reducing feelings of loneliness and isolation.

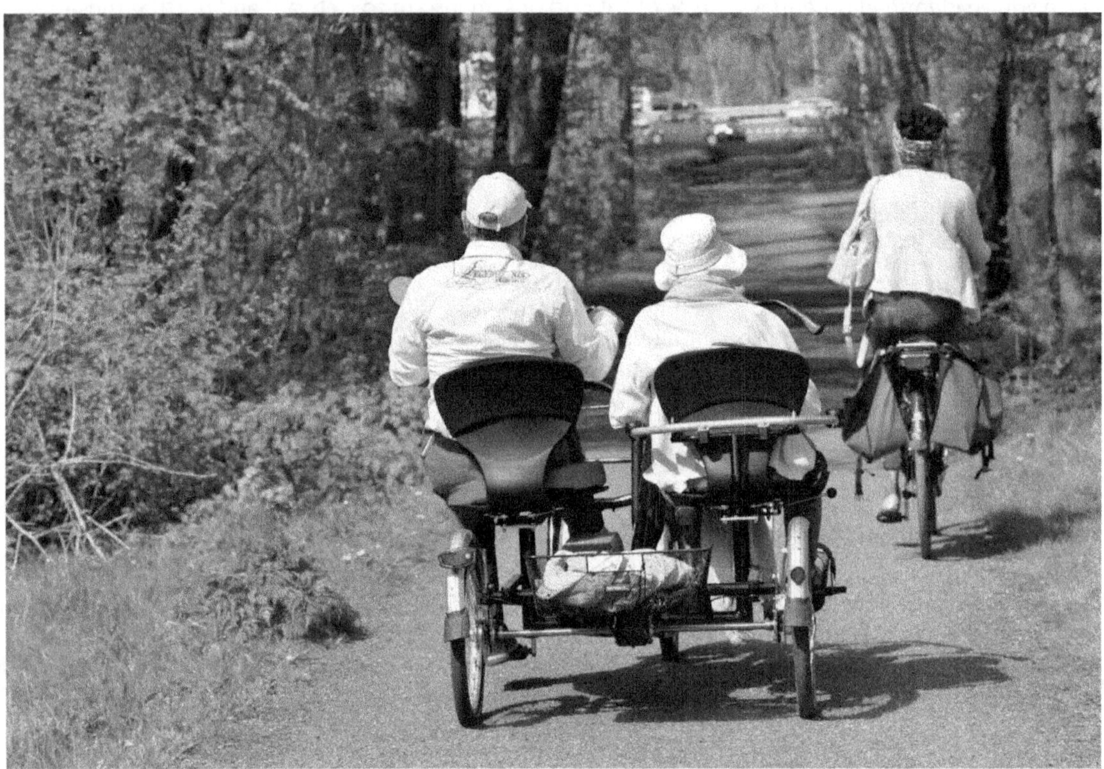

Additionally, social support provides practical assistance and resources when needed. Whether it's helping with daily tasks, offering advice or guidance, or providing financial or logistical support, having a supportive network of friends, family, or colleagues can lighten the burden of stress and help navigate through difficult situations more effectively.

Moreover, social support fosters a sense of belonging and connection, which is essential for mental and emotional well-being. Feeling connected to others and having meaningful relationships contributes to feelings of happiness, fulfillment, and overall life satisfaction.

Furthermore, social support can positively impact physical health outcomes. Studies have shown that individuals with strong social connections tend to have lower rates of chronic diseases, faster recovery times from illness or injury, and overall better health outcomes compared to those who are socially isolated.

In summary, social support is essential for promoting resilience, happiness, and well-being. Cultivating meaningful relationships and building a supportive network of friends, family, and colleagues can provide emotional encouragement, practical assistance, and a sense of belonging that enhances overall quality of life.

9.2 Finding Accountability Partners

Finding accountability partners is a valuable strategy for achieving goals and staying on track with personal development endeavors. An accountability partner is someone who holds you responsible for your actions, provides support, and helps you stay focused on your goals.

One way to find accountability partners is to look within your existing network of friends, family, or colleagues. Consider individuals who share similar goals or aspirations and who you trust to provide honest feedback and encouragement.

Additionally, you can join online communities, forums, or social media groups dedicated to specific interests or goals. These platforms provide opportunities to connect with like-minded individuals who can serve as accountability partners, offering support, motivation, and accountability.

Furthermore, consider seeking out professional accountability partners, such as coaches, mentors, or therapists, who can provide expert guidance and support tailored to your specific needs and goals.

When choosing accountability partners, it's essential to establish clear expectations and communication channels. Clearly define your goals, timelines, and the level of accountability you're seeking, and regularly check in with your accountability partners to discuss progress, challenges, and strategies for overcoming obstacles.

By finding accountability partners who are invested in your success, you can increase motivation, stay accountable to your goals, and achieve greater success in your personal development journey.

9.3 Seeking Professional Support

Seeking professional support is a proactive step towards addressing challenges, achieving goals, and fostering personal growth. Professional support encompasses seeking guidance, expertise, and assistance from individuals who possess specialized knowledge and experience in a particular field or area of expertise.

One common form of professional support is therapy or counseling, where individuals seek the help of trained mental health professionals to address issues such as anxiety, depression, trauma, or relationship problems. Therapists provide a safe and supportive environment for individuals to explore their thoughts, feelings, and behaviors, and develop coping strategies and solutions to overcome challenges.

Additionally, seeking professional support may involve hiring coaches, mentors, or consultants who can provide expert guidance and accountability in specific areas of interest or goals. Coaches and mentors offer personalized guidance, feedback, and encouragement to help individuals clarify their goals, overcome obstacles, and achieve greater success in their personal or professional lives.

Furthermore, professionals such as financial advisors, career counselors, or nutritionists can provide valuable expertise and support in areas related to financial planning, career development, or health and wellness.

Overall, seeking professional support empowers individuals to address challenges, gain valuable insights, and make positive changes in their lives. Whether it's therapy, coaching, or consulting, professional support offers a valuable resource for personal growth, self-improvement, and achieving greater fulfillment and success.

Chapter 10: Long-Term Maintenance

Long-term maintenance is a critical phase in any journey of personal development, whether it's maintaining a healthy lifestyle, managing weight, or sustaining progress in career or personal goals. It involves establishing sustainable habits, routines, and strategies to ensure continued success and prevent regression over time.

One key aspect of long-term maintenance is consistency. Maintaining consistency in healthy habits such as regular exercise, balanced nutrition, and self-care practices is essential for sustaining progress and preventing relapse. Consistency helps solidify habits into routines and ensures that positive behaviors become ingrained into daily life.

Additionally, long-term maintenance requires ongoing monitoring and adjustment. Regularly assessing progress, identifying areas for improvement, and making necessary adjustments to routines or strategies helps to adapt to changing circumstances and prevent stagnation. This may involve setting new goals, trying new approaches, or seeking support when needed.

Furthermore, cultivating a positive mindset and resilience is crucial for long-term maintenance. Recognizing that setbacks are a natural part of the journey and viewing challenges as opportunities for growth helps maintain motivation and perseverance during difficult times. Building resilience allows individuals to bounce back from setbacks and stay committed to their long-term goals despite obstacles.

Moreover, establishing a strong support system is vital for long-term maintenance. Surrounding oneself with supportive friends, family, mentors, or peers who encourage and hold accountable can provide invaluable motivation and reinforcement during the maintenance phase.

Finally, prioritizing self-care and stress management is essential for sustaining long-term success. Taking time for rest, relaxation, and activities that promote mental and emotional well-being helps prevent burnout and maintain balance in life.

In summary, long-term maintenance requires a combination of consistency, monitoring, adjustment, resilience, support, and self-care. By establishing sustainable habits, staying adaptable, fostering a positive mindset, and prioritizing self-care, individuals can sustain progress and achieve lasting success in their personal development journey.

10.1 Transitioning to Maintenance

Transitioning to maintenance is a crucial phase in any journey of personal development, whether it's weight loss, fitness, career advancement, or personal growth. It marks the shift from actively pursuing goals to sustaining progress and preventing regression over the long term.

During this phase, individuals begin to adjust their focus from achieving specific milestones to establishing sustainable habits and routines that support continued success. This involves consolidating the progress made during the active phase and incorporating strategies to maintain achievements in the long run.

Transitioning to maintenance requires a shift in mindset towards sustainability and balance. Rather than solely focusing on strict adherence to goals or restrictions, individuals prioritize flexibility, moderation, and self-awareness. This allows for more freedom in lifestyle choices while still maintaining progress and preventing setbacks.

Moreover, individuals in the maintenance phase continue to monitor their progress, albeit with less intensity than during the active phase. Regularly assessing behaviors, outcomes, and challenges helps identify areas for improvement and make necessary adjustments to routines or strategies.

Overall, transitioning to maintenance is about embracing a lifestyle that supports long-term success and well-being. By establishing sustainable habits, maintaining balance, and staying mindful of progress, individuals can sustain their achievements and continue to thrive in their personal development journey.

10.2 Strategies for Preventing Weight Regain

Preventing weight regain is a critical aspect of long-term weight management and involves implementing strategies that support sustainable lifestyle changes. One key strategy is to focus on gradual, sustainable weight loss rather than quick fixes or crash diets. Sustainable weight loss involves making gradual changes to eating habits and physical activity levels that can be maintained over the long term.

Another effective strategy is to prioritize balanced nutrition by including a variety of nutrient-dense foods in your diet, such as fruits, vegetables, lean proteins, and whole grains. Balancing macronutrients and controlling portion sizes can help prevent overeating and promote feelings of fullness and satisfaction.

Regular physical activity is also essential for weight maintenance. Incorporating both cardiovascular exercise and strength training into your routine can help burn calories, build muscle mass, and boost metabolism, making it easier to maintain weight loss over time.

Additionally, monitoring progress and staying accountable can help prevent weight regain. Keeping track of food intake, physical activity, and body measurements can help identify potential triggers for weight regain and allow for adjustments to be made as needed.

Finally, cultivating a supportive environment and mindset is crucial for long-term success. Surrounding yourself with supportive friends, family, or peers who encourage healthy habits and provide accountability can help reinforce positive behaviors and reduce the risk of relapse.

Additionally, practicing self-compassion and resilience can help navigate setbacks and challenges along the way. By implementing these strategies, individuals can prevent weight regain and maintain their progress towards long-term health and wellness goals.

10.3 Making Health a Lifestyle

Making health a lifestyle involves adopting habits and behaviors that prioritize physical, mental, and emotional well-being as integral parts of daily life. Rather than viewing health as a temporary pursuit or short-term goal, it entails cultivating sustainable practices that support long-term vitality and overall quality of life.

At the core of making health a lifestyle is a commitment to balanced nutrition, regular physical activity, and adequate rest and relaxation. This includes choosing nutrient-dense foods, staying hydrated, and engaging in regular exercise that promotes cardiovascular health, strength, and flexibility.

Moreover, making health a lifestyle extends beyond physical health to encompass mental and emotional well-being. This involves managing stress effectively, practicing mindfulness and self-care, and nurturing supportive relationships that contribute to overall happiness and fulfillment.

Additionally, making health a lifestyle requires ongoing self-awareness and self-reflection. It involves listening to your body's cues, honoring your unique needs and preferences, and making choices that align with your values and goals.

Ultimately, making health a lifestyle is about embracing a holistic approach to well-being that integrates healthy habits into all aspects of daily life. By prioritizing health as a central value and consistently practicing behaviors that support vitality and longevity, individuals can enjoy lasting benefits and a higher quality of life.

Chapter 11: Setting Realistic Goals

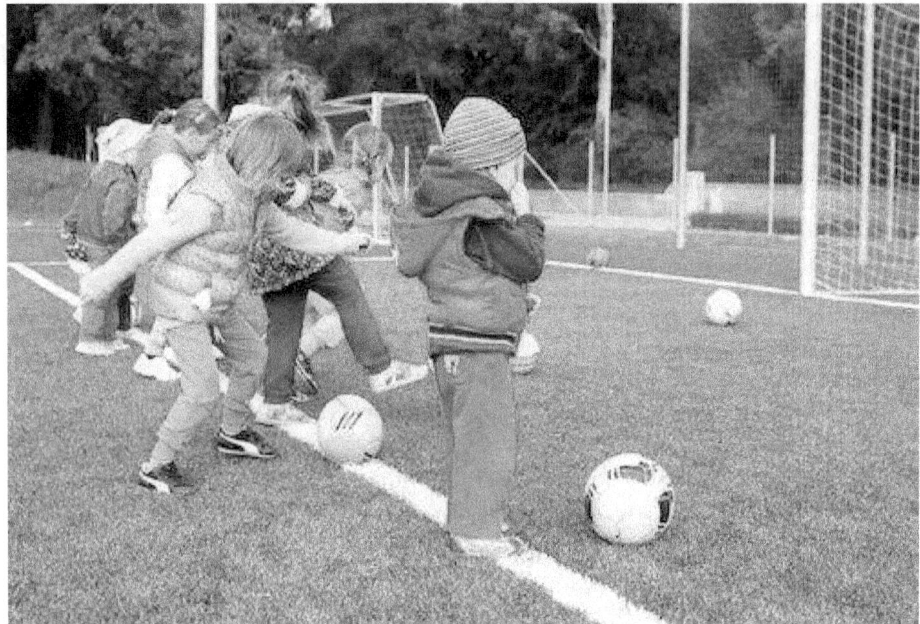

Setting realistic and achievable goals is crucial for long-term success. Rather than focusing solely on a specific number on the scale, consider setting goals related to behavior changes and lifestyle improvements.

For example, aim to incorporate more fruits and vegetables into your diet, commit to regular physical activity, or prioritize getting an adequate amount of sleep each night. These small, actionable goals can add up to significant improvements in your overall health and weight over time.

Setting goals is a vital aspect of both personal and professional development, but they must also be realistic. Unrealistic objectives can cause irritation, disappointment, and even the complete abandoning of the goal-setting process. Here are some important ideas to bear in mind when developing realistic goals:

1. Define Specific and Clear Goals

Establish a clear goal. Vague goals such as "lose weight" or "get in shape" are less effective than precise goals like "lose 10 pounds in three months" or "run a 5k race in six weeks." Specific goals provide clarity and direction, making it easier to strive toward.

Specific and clear goals are essential for guiding individuals or organizations towards desired outcomes with clarity and precision. These goals are characterized by their specificity, outlining precisely what needs to be accomplished, and clarity, ensuring that the objective is well-defined and easily understandable. When setting specific and clear goals, several key elements should be considered:

1.Measurable:

Goals should be quantifiable, allowing progress to be tracked and evaluated objectively. This could involve metrics such as numbers, percentages, or specific milestones.

2. Attainable:

Goals should be realistic and achievable within the given resources and constraints. Setting unattainable goals can lead to frustration and demotivation.

3. Relevant:

Goals should align with the broader objectives and mission of the individual or organization. They should contribute meaningfully to overall success and progress.

4. Time-bound:

Goals should have a clearly defined timeframe for completion. This helps create urgency and accountability, preventing procrastination and ensuring timely progress.

5. Clear and concise:

Goals should be articulated in a straightforward manner, avoiding ambiguity or confusion. Everyone involved should have a clear understanding of what is expected.

Overall, specific and clear goals provide a roadmap for action, guiding decision-making, motivating individuals, and fostering accountability. They serve as a foundation for effective planning, execution, and ultimately, achievement.

2. Evaluate Your Resources and Limitations:

Evaluate your resources, including time, energy, cash, and support systems. Setting goals that need more resources than you have may set you up for failure. Be realistic about what you can do given your existing circumstances.

Evaluating resources and limitations is a crucial step in any endeavor, whether it's an individual pursuing personal goals or an organization striving for success. This evaluation involves assessing the assets, capabilities, and constraints that will influence the ability to achieve objectives effectively. Here are some key considerations:

1. Financial Resources:
   Assessing the available budget and financial resources is essential. This includes funds for investment, operational expenses, and potential sources of revenue or funding.
2. Human Capital:
   Evaluating the skills, expertise, and capacity of personnel is vital. Understanding the strengths and weaknesses of the team enables effective resource allocation and talent management.
3. Technological Infrastructure:
   Considering the technological tools, equipment, and systems available is critical. This includes hardware, software, communication networks, and any other technological resources required to support operations.
4. Physical Assets:
   Evaluating physical assets such as facilities, equipment, and inventory provides insights into operational capabilities and potential limitations.
5. Time Constraints:
   Understanding deadlines, timeframes, and project schedules is essential. Time constraints can impact planning, execution, and overall project success.
6. Regulatory and Legal Considerations:

Assessing compliance requirements, regulations, and legal constraints is necessary. Failure to adhere to applicable laws and regulations can result in significant setbacks or penalties.

By thoroughly evaluating resources and limitations, individuals and organizations can make informed decisions, allocate resources effectively, and mitigate risks. This process lays the groundwork for strategic planning and successful execution of objectives.

3. Break Goals Down into Smaller Steps:

Large goals can be intimidating, leading to delay or avoidance. Break down enormous ambitions into smaller, more achievable chunks. This not only makes the objective more attainable, but it also gives you a sense of accomplishment and momentum as you check off each step.

Breaking goals down into smaller steps is a fundamental strategy for effective planning and execution. This approach, often referred to as "chunking" or "task decomposition," involves dividing larger, overarching goals into smaller, more manageable tasks or milestones. Here's why it's essential and how to do it effectively:

1. Clarity and Focus:
   Breaking goals into smaller steps provides clarity on what needs to be done and helps individuals or teams stay focused on actionable tasks.
2. Progress Tracking:
   Smaller steps make it easier to track progress and measure success incrementally. This allows for adjustments and course corrections along the way.
3. Motivation and Momentum:
   Achieving smaller milestones provides a sense of accomplishment and motivation, fueling momentum towards larger goals.
4. Risk Mitigation:
   Breaking goals down helps identify potential risks or challenges early on, allowing for proactive problem-solving and risk mitigation strategies.
5. Resource Allocation:
   Smaller steps facilitate more efficient resource allocation, as tasks can be prioritized based on their importance and dependencies.

To break goals down effectively:

- Start by identifying the overarching goal or objective.
- Divide it into smaller, manageable tasks or milestones.
- Prioritize these tasks based on urgency, importance, and dependencies.
- Assign responsibilities and deadlines for each task.
- Regularly review progress and adjust the plan as needed.

By breaking goals down into smaller steps, individuals and teams can increase their chances of success by making complex objectives more achievable and manageable. It's a practical approach that promotes clarity, progress, and ultimately, goal attainment.

4. Create a Timeline that is Realistic:

Consider how much time you will actually need to attain your objectives. Rushing to attain a goal in an unsustainable timeline might result in burnout or a sacrifice of quality.

A too-long timescale, on the other hand, may lead to complacency. Set deadlines that are both challenging and feasible in order to strike a balance.

Creating a realistic timeline is essential for effective goal planning and execution. A timeline outlines the sequence of activities and deadlines required to achieve specific objectives within a predetermined timeframe. Here are some key considerations for creating a realistic timeline:

1. Assess Available Resources:
   Before creating a timeline, assess the resources available, including human resources, financial resources, and technological capabilities. Consider any constraints or limitations that may affect the timeline, such as budget constraints or availability of skilled personnel.
2. Break Goals into Smaller Tasks:
   As mentioned earlier, breaking goals down into smaller, manageable tasks is crucial. Use these smaller tasks to populate the timeline, ensuring each task is assigned a realistic timeframe for completion.
3. Consider Dependencies and Constraints:
   Identify any dependencies between tasks and any constraints that may impact the timeline. This could include waiting for approvals, coordinating with external stakeholders, or relying on specific resources or technologies.
4. Build in Buffer Time:
   It's important to build in buffer time or contingency allowances to account for unforeseen delays or setbacks. This helps mitigate risks and ensures that the timeline remains realistic even in the face of unexpected challenges.
5. Regularly Review and Adjust:
   Continuously monitor progress against the timeline and be prepared to adjust as needed. If tasks are taking longer than anticipated or priorities shift, be flexible in adapting the timeline accordingly.
6. Communicate and Collaborate:
   Ensure that all stakeholders are aware of the timeline and their respective responsibilities. Foster open communication and collaboration to address any issues or concerns that may arise.

By creating a realistic timeline, individuals and teams can effectively plan and execute their goals, increasing the likelihood of success while minimizing the risk of delays or failure. It provides a roadmap for progress, keeps everyone accountable, and helps maintain focus and momentum towards achieving desired outcomes.

5. Maintain your flexibility and adaptability

Life is unpredictable, and circumstances can shift along the road. Be prepared to change your goals and techniques as needed. Flexibility permits you to adjust to new problems or opportunities without jeopardizing your ultimate goals.

Maintaining flexibility and adaptability is crucial when working towards goals, as unforeseen circumstances and changing environments are inevitable. Here are some key reasons why it's essential and how to effectively incorporate flexibility into goal pursuit:

1. Responding to Change:
   Flexibility allows individuals and teams to respond effectively to changes in circumstances, such as unexpected challenges, new opportunities, or shifting priorities. Being adaptable enables quick adjustments to plans and strategies to stay on course towards the goal.
2. Embracing Innovation:
   Flexibility fosters an environment where new ideas and innovative approaches can be explored. It encourages creativity and experimentation, leading to potential breakthroughs and improved outcomes.
3. Navigating Uncertainty:
   In dynamic and uncertain environments, maintaining flexibility helps navigate ambiguity and volatility. It allows for agile decision-making and course corrections based on emerging information or evolving conditions.
4. Maximizing Resilience:
   Flexibility builds resilience, enabling individuals and teams to bounce back from setbacks or failures. It fosters a mindset of learning and growth, turning challenges into opportunities for improvement and adaptation.

To maintain flexibility and adaptability:

- Stay Open-Minded: Remain open to new ideas, feedback, and alternative approaches. Embrace change as an opportunity for growth and improvement.
- Be Agile: Foster a culture of agility by encouraging quick decision-making, iterative progress, and continuous learning.
- Communicate Effectively: Keep lines of communication open among team members, stakeholders, and partners. Regularly assess progress and discuss potential adjustments as needed.
- Empowerment and Autonomy: Encourage autonomy and empower individuals to make decisions and take ownership of their work. Provide support and resources to facilitate adaptability.

By maintaining flexibility and adaptability, individuals and teams can navigate challenges, capitalize on opportunities, and ultimately, achieve their goals more effectively in dynamic and evolving environments.

5. Recognize progress:

Recognize and applaud any improvement you make, no matter how tiny. Recognizing your accomplishments boosts your drive and confidence, helping you stay on course to reach your larger goals.

You set yourself up for success by defining realistic, detailed, resource-conserving goals that are broken down into manageable steps and flexible to change.

A too-long timescale, on the other hand, may lead to complacency. Set deadlines that are both challenging and feasible in order to strike a balance.

Recognizing progress is vital for maintaining motivation, boosting morale, and sustaining momentum towards achieving goals. Here are several reasons why acknowledging progress is crucial and how it can be effectively implemented:

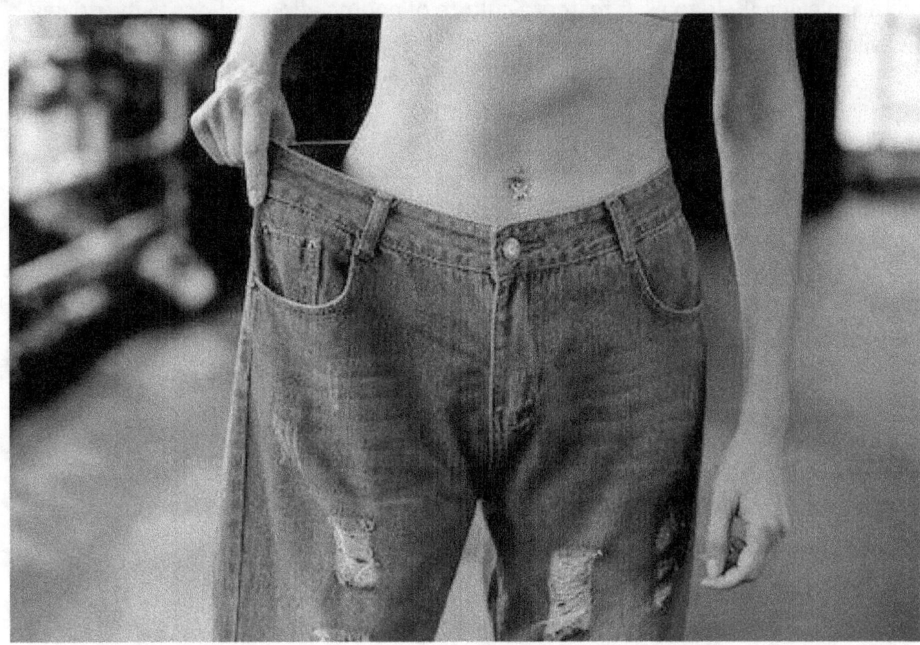

1. Motivation and Engagement:
    Celebrating progress provides a sense of accomplishment and reinforces motivation. Recognizing achievements, no matter how small, encourages individuals to continue their efforts and stay engaged in the pursuit of their goals.
2. Positive Reinforcement:
    Recognizing progress reinforces positive behaviors and actions. It acknowledges the effort and dedication put forth by individuals or teams, reinforcing their commitment to the goal.
3. Boosting Confidence:
    Acknowledging progress helps build confidence and self-esteem. When individuals see evidence of their progress, they feel more capable and confident in their abilities, which can drive further success.
4. Fostering Team Spirit:
    Recognizing progress fosters a sense of camaraderie and teamwork. It acknowledges the collective effort of the team and strengthens bonds among team members, promoting collaboration and a shared sense of purpose.

To effectively recognize progress:

- Set Milestones: Establish clear milestones or checkpoints along the journey towards the goal. Celebrate reaching these milestones to acknowledge progress and keep morale high.
- Provide Feedback: Offer constructive feedback and praise for achievements. Recognize individual contributions and highlight areas of improvement to encourage continuous growth.
- Celebrate Successes: Take time to celebrate significant achievements or milestones. This could involve team celebrations, rewards, or recognition ceremonies to commemorate progress and success.

- Regular Check-ins: Conduct regular check-ins to review progress and provide recognition. Acknowledge both individual and collective accomplishments to reinforce a positive culture of recognition.

By consistently recognizing progress, individuals and teams are more likely to stay motivated, focused, and committed to achieving their goals. It fosters a culture of appreciation and positivity, driving ongoing success and growth.

Nutritional Strategies

A balanced and nutritious diet is critical for obtaining and maintaining your target weight. Consider the following nutritional ideas to help you lose weight:

Nutritional strategies play a crucial role in promoting overall health and well-being by providing the body with essential nutrients necessary for optimal functioning. Here are several key aspects of effective nutritional strategies:

1. Balanced Diet:
   A balanced diet includes a variety of foods from all food groups, such as fruits, vegetables, whole grains, lean proteins, and healthy fats. This ensures adequate intake of essential nutrients, vitamins, and minerals necessary for energy production, immune function, and maintenance of bodily functions.
2. Portion Control:
   Managing portion sizes is important to prevent overeating and maintain a healthy weight. Portion control helps regulate calorie intake and can contribute to better weight management and overall health.
3. Hydration:
   Staying hydrated is essential for proper bodily function, including digestion, nutrient absorption, and temperature regulation. Drinking an adequate amount of water throughout the day is important for overall health and well-being.
4. Mindful Eating:
   Practicing mindful eating involves paying attention to hunger cues, eating slowly, and savoring each bite. This helps prevent overeating, promotes better digestion, and enhances the enjoyment of food.
5. Meal Planning:
   Planning meals ahead of time can help ensure balanced nutrition and prevent reliance on unhealthy convenience foods. Meal planning allows for healthier food choices and can save time and money.
6. Supplementation:
   In some cases, supplementation may be necessary to address specific nutrient deficiencies or to support overall health. However, it's important to consult with a healthcare professional before starting any supplementation regimen.

Overall, adopting a balanced and mindful approach to nutrition is essential for promoting health, preventing chronic diseases, and supporting overall well-being. By incorporating these nutritional strategies into daily life, individuals can optimize their health and quality of life.

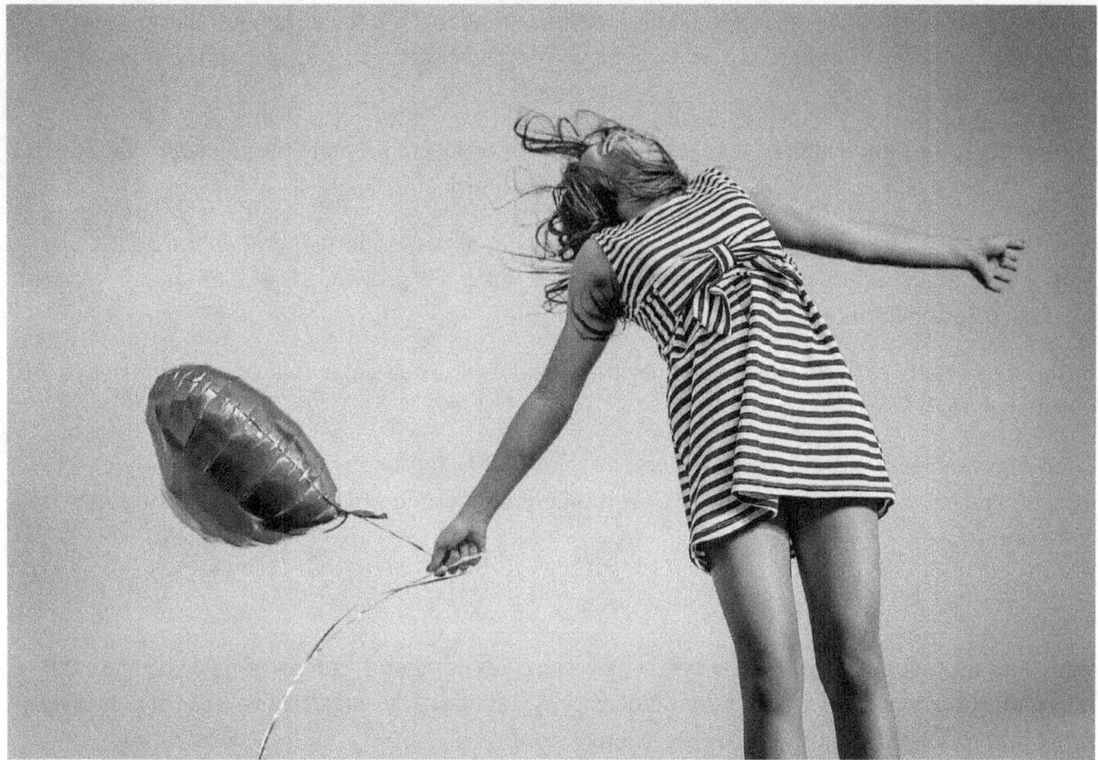

Nutrition is extremely important for our general health and well-being. Adopting good eating methods can help us maintain a healthy weight, promote optimal bodily functions, and lower our risk of chronic diseases. Here are some basic guidelines to help you achieve better nutrition and a healthy lifestyle:

1. Focus on Whole Foods:

Focus your diet on whole, unprocessed foods including fruits, vegetables, whole grains, lean meats, and healthy fats. These foods are nutrient dense, containing vital vitamins, minerals, fibre, and antioxidants that support overall health.

Whole foods are an important part of a healthy eating plan. Whole foods are little processed and retain their inherent ingredients, which provide several health benefits.

Whole foods include fruits and vegetables, whole grains, lean proteins, and healthy fats, all of which contain vital vitamins, minerals, fibre, and antioxidants.

Prioritizing whole foods in your diet provides your body with the nutrients it requires to thrive, promotes maximum health, and lowers the risk of chronic diseases.

Incorporating whole foods into your meals enhances satiety, aids weight management, and encourages a balanced and sustainable approach to nutrition in the long run.

2. Balance the Macronutrients:

Aim for a carbohydrate, protein, and fat balance in your meals. Carbohydrates give energy, proteins promote muscle repair and growth, while lipids are necessary for cell structure and hormone manufacturing.

Choose complex carbohydrates, lean proteins, and healthy fats to promote overall health and satiety. A well-rounded diet requires careful attention to macronutrient balance.

Macronutrients, which include carbs, proteins, and lipids, all play important roles in the body. Carbohydrates give energy, proteins promote muscle repair and growth, while lipids are necessary for cell structure and hormone manufacturing.

By having a variety of these macronutrients in your meals, you guarantee that your body receives the nutrition it need for optimal operation.

Choosing complex carbohydrates, lean proteins, and healthy fats improves long-term energy, muscular development, and overall health and satiety, supporting a balanced and satisfying approach to eating.

3. Practice Portion Control:

To avoid overeating, limit your meal sizes. Use visual clues or measuring tools to help you learn the proper portion proportions for different food groups. Eating slowly and attentively can also assist to avoid overconsumption and improve digestion.

Portion control is essential for following a healthy diet. It entails being careful of serving amounts in order to prevent overeating and aid with weight management. Understanding optimal portion sizes for different food types will help you avoid ingesting too many calories and better regulate your intake. Eating slowly and deliberately, using visual cues or measuring instruments, and being aware of hunger and fullness cues all help to improve portion management.

By exercising portion management, you can eat a balanced diet while indulging in your favourite foods in moderation, resulting in better overall health and well-being.

4. Stay Hydrated.

Drink plenty of water throughout the day to keep yourself hydrated. Water is necessary for maintaining body temperature, assisting digestion, and carrying nutrients and oxygen to cells. To stay hydrated, limit sugary beverages and instead drink water, herbal teas, or infused water.

Staying hydrated is critical for your overall health and well-being. Water is essential for maintaining body temperature, assisting digestion, and moving nutrients throughout the body.

Maintaining correct hydration levels helps to prevent dehydration, which can cause fatigue, headaches, and impaired cognitive function.

Aim to drink plenty of water throughout the day, especially during physical activity or in hot weather. Herbal teas and infused water are also great hydration options.

Prioritizing hydration helps to maintain optimal biological processes, increase energy levels, and promote overall health and vitality.

5. Add Variety and Color:

Include a variety of colored fruits and vegetables in your meals to ensure you obtain a wide range of nutrients. Different colors represent different nutrients, so try to eat a variety of fruits and vegetables every day.

Including variety and color in your diet is essential for optimal nutrition. Different colored fruits and vegetables offer a diverse range of vitamins, minerals, and antioxidants, each contributing to your overall health in unique ways.

Aim to incorporate a rainbow of colors into your meals, such as red tomatoes, orange carrots, green spinach, and purple berries.

By diversifying your food choices, you ensure that you receive a wide array of nutrients that support immune function, heart health, digestion, and more. Embrace variety and color to nourish your body and enjoy a vibrant, well-balanced diet.

6. Plan and Prepare Meals:

Take time to plan and prepare your meals in advance to ensure they're balanced and nutritious. Batch cooking, meal prepping, and using healthy cooking methods such as steaming, baking, or grilling can help you stay on track with your nutrition goals.

Planning and preparing meals ahead of time is an important part of eating a healthy and balanced diet. By planning your meals ahead of time, you can make sure you have nutritious options on hand and avoid depending on unhealthy convenience items.

Batch cooking, meal preparing, and developing a weekly meal plan can assist to streamline the cooking process and save time during hectic weekdays. Furthermore, meal planning allows you to make healthier choices, control portion sizes, and minimize food waste.

By incorporating meal planning and preparation into your daily routine, you will be better able to achieve your nutrition objectives.

Pay attention to your own body

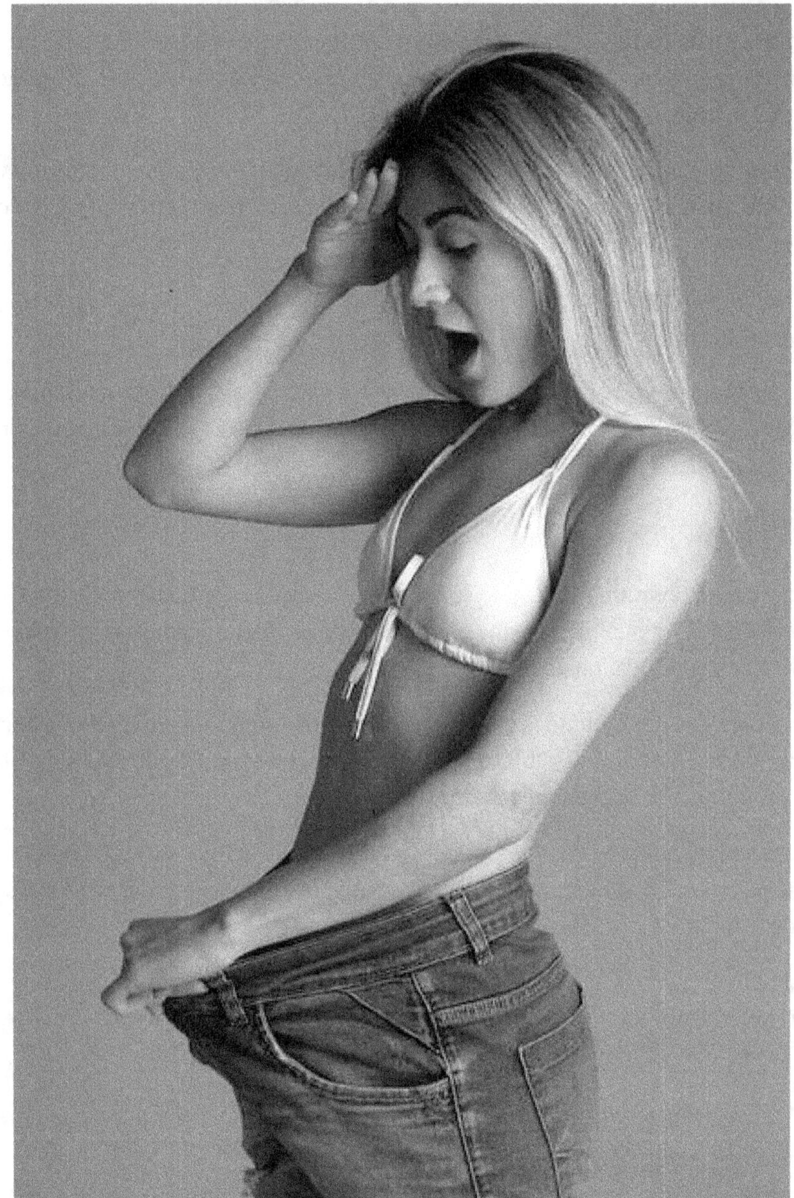

Pay attention to hunger and fullness cues, eating when you're hungry and stopping when you're full. Avoid tight diets and overly strict regulations in favor of fueling your body with nutritious foods that make you feel good.

Listening to your body is critical for establishing a positive connection with food and boosting your overall health.

Pay attention to hunger and fullness cues, eating when you're hungry and finishing when you're full. Tuning in to your body's signals might help you avoid overeating and promote mindful eating.

Consider how different foods make you feel. Consider how certain foods energize you, while others make you feel sluggish or bloated. By acknowledging your body's requirements and preferences, you can make informed decisions that benefit your health and foster a happy connection with food. Trust your body's wisdom and feed it appropriately.

Adopting these nutrition techniques will help you develop good eating habits that benefit your overall health and contribute to a lively and meaningful lifestyle. Remember that even little changes might result in major gains to your health over time.

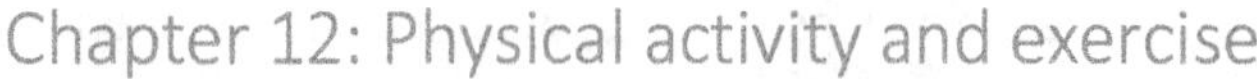

Chapter 12: Physical activity and exercise

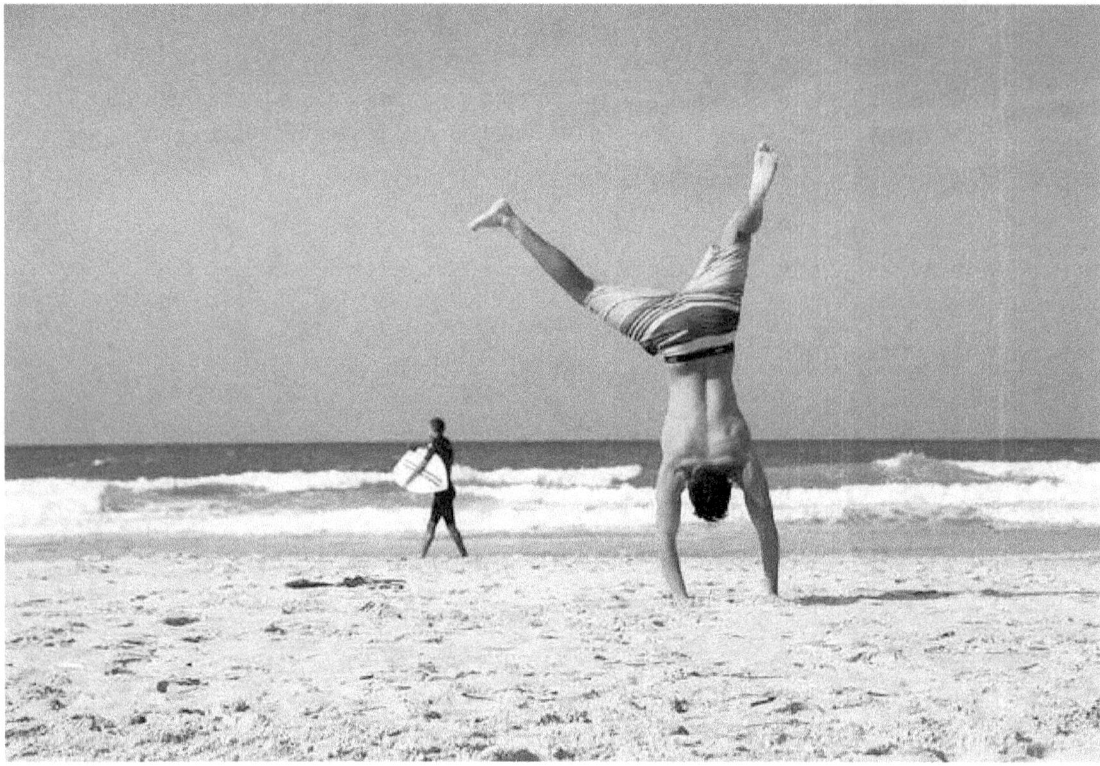

Physical activity and exercise play an important role in health and well-being.

Physical activity and exercise are essential for improving overall health and well-being. Regular physical activity has numerous benefits for both the body and the mind, including improving cardiovascular health, enhancing mood, and lowering the risk of chronic diseases.

In this post, we will look at the benefits of physical activity and exercise, as well as how to incorporate them into your daily routine.

Importance of Physical Activity

1. Improves Cardiovascular Health:

Regular physical activity, such as brisk walking, jogging, or cycling, helps to strengthen the heart and improve circulation. It reduces blood pressure, cholesterol levels, and the risk of heart disease and stroke.

Improved cardiovascular health is a foundational component of overall well-being, and regular physical exercise is critical in reaching and maintaining it.

Brisk walking, running, cycling, swimming, and dancing all help to strengthen the heart muscle, increase circulation, and improve cardiovascular health.

Exercise lowers blood pressure and cholesterol levels by boosting heart rate and blood flow, therefore lowering the risk of heart disease and stroke.

Furthermore, frequent physical exercise encourages blood vessel dilatation, which increases their flexibility and effectiveness in transporting oxygen and nutrients to tissues throughout the body.

Exercise not only has a direct impact on cardiovascular health, but it also helps with weight management, which is another important aspect of heart health.

Maintaining a healthy body weight through regular physical activity puts less burden on the heart and minimizes the risk of obesity-related illnesses including type 2 diabetes and metabolic syndrome.

Overall, including regular exercise into your daily routine is an excellent approach to improve cardiovascular health, improve circulation, lower blood pressure and cholesterol levels, and minimize your risk of heart disease and stroke.

Prioritizing physical activity will provide you with the benefits of a stronger, healthier heart and a longer, more vibrant life.

2. Weight Management

Physical activity is important for weight management since it burns calories and boosts metabolism. It promotes a healthy body weight and prevents obesity, which is linked to a variety of health problems such as type 2 diabetes, high blood pressure, and some malignancies.

Weight management is an important part of general health and well-being, and it includes both obtaining and maintaining a healthy body weight.

It entails striking a balance between energy intake (calories consumed) and energy expenditure (calories used for physical activity and metabolic activities).

To effectively manage weight, a comprehensive approach is required, which includes healthy eating habits, frequent physical activity, appropriate sleep, stress management, and a supportive environment. Including full, nutrient-dense foods in your diet,

Such as fruits, vegetables, lean meats, and whole grains, can help control appetite, regulate metabolism, and offer necessary nutrients while minimizing processed meals, sugary beverages, and excessive calorie consumption.

Regular physical activity plays a vital role in weight management by burning calories, building muscle mass, and boosting metabolism. Aim for a combination of cardiovascular exercise, strength training, and flexibility exercises to support overall fitness and weight loss efforts.

Additionally, maintaining a consistent sleep schedule, managing stress levels, and surrounding yourself with a supportive social network can all contribute to successful weight management.

By adopting healthy lifestyle habits and making sustainable changes over time, you can achieve and maintain a healthy body weight, improve overall health, and reduce the risk of obesity-related conditions such as diabetes, heart disease, and certain cancers.

3. Improved mental health:

Exercise has a strong impact on mental health, helping to alleviate feelings of anxiety, sadness, and stress. Physical activity causes the production of endorphins, neurotransmitters that increase feelings of enjoyment and relaxation, resulting in a better mood and mental clarity.

One of the major advantages of regular physical activity and exercise is improved mental health. Exercise has been proved to have a significant impact on mental health by reducing feelings of anxiety, depression, and stress.

When you exercise, your body releases endorphins, neurotransmitters that act as natural mood lifters and pain relievers. These endorphins create a feeling of euphoria and relaxation, often referred to as the "runner's high."

Regular physical activity also stimulates the production of serotonin and dopamine, neurotransmitters that regulate mood, emotions, and motivation.

Moreover, exercise serves as a healthy coping mechanism for stress and anxiety. Physical activity reduces levels of cortisol, the body's stress hormone, and promotes relaxation, leading to a calmer state of mind.

Additionally, the focus and concentration required during exercise can distract from negative thoughts and worries, providing a temporary respite from daily stressors.

Furthermore, regular exercise can improve self-esteem and body image, fostering a positive outlook on life. As you achieve fitness goals and experience improvements in strength, endurance, and overall health, you gain a sense of accomplishment and confidence in your abilities.

In summary, incorporating regular physical activity and exercise into your routine is not only beneficial for your physical health but also for your mental well-being.

By reducing symptoms of anxiety, depression, and stress, exercise helps promote emotional resilience, enhance mood, and improve overall quality of life.

4. Increased Muscle and Bone Strength:

Weight-bearing activities such as strength training, resistance exercises, and weightlifting serve to develop muscle strength and bone density. This not only improves physical performance, but also lowers the risk of osteoporosis and fractures, especially in older persons.

Strengthening muscles and bones is an important element of general health, and regular exercise can help you achieve it. Strength training, resistance exercises, and weight-bearing activities are very helpful at improving muscle and bone strength.

Strength training involves challenging and strengthening muscles through the use of resistance, such as free weights, resistance bands, or bodyweight exercises.

Muscle growth, physical strength, and endurance can all be enhanced by gradually increasing resistance over time. Strong muscles not only aid with posture and balance, but they also help to prevent injuries and improve overall mobility and function.

Weight-bearing activities like walking, running, hiking, and dancing also support bone health by encouraging bone growth and density. Weight-bearing workouts stress bones, causing them to adapt and get stronger over time. This is particularly crucial for avoiding osteoporosis and lowering the risk of fractures in older persons.

Furthermore, strong muscles help to maintain healthy joints and increase general stability, lowering the chance of falls and injuries.

Strength training and weight-bearing activities can help you create and maintain stronger muscles and bones, resulting in better physical performance, a higher quality of life, and a longer lifespan.

5. Better Sleep Quality:

Regular physical activity can improve sleep quality and duration, leading to more restful nights and increased daytime alertness. It helps regulate circadian rhythms and reduces symptoms of insomnia, promoting overall sleep hygiene.

Improving sleep quality is a crucial aspect of overall health and well-being, and regular physical activity plays a significant role in achieving this goal. Engaging in regular exercise has been shown to promote better sleep by enhancing both the quantity and quality of restorative sleep.

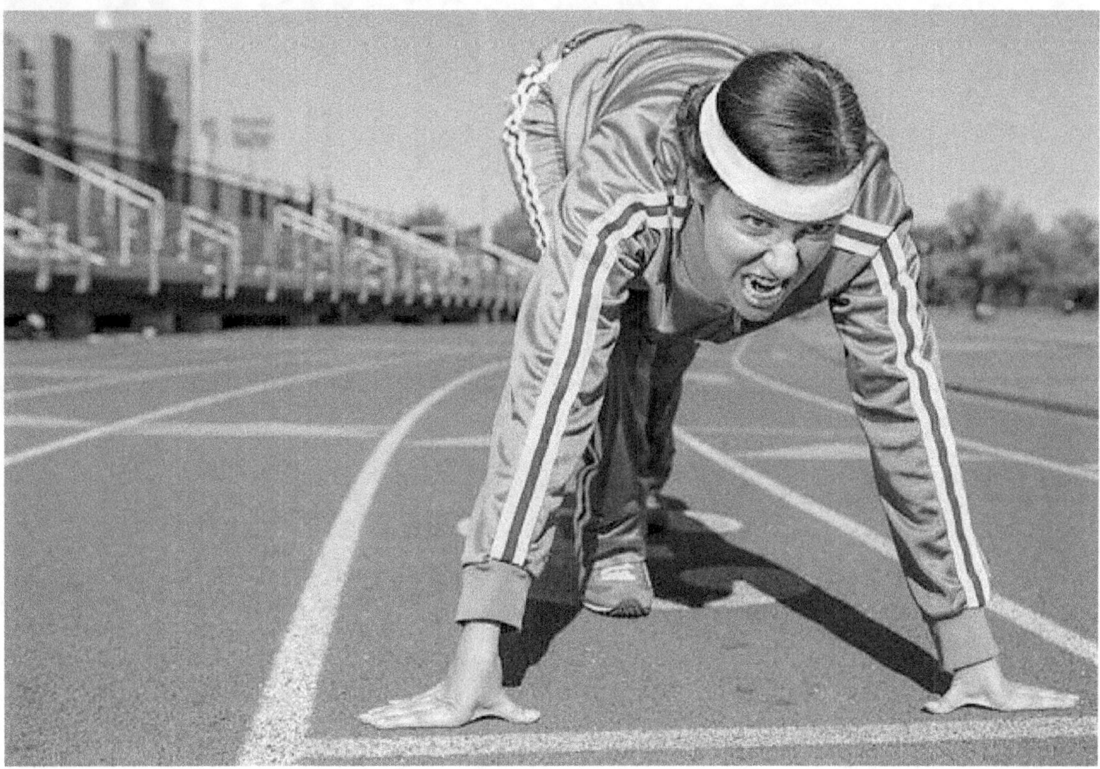

Exercise helps regulate the body's internal clock, known as the circadian rhythm, which controls the sleep-wake cycle. By exposing the body to natural daylight and physical activity during the day, and promoting relaxation in the evening, exercise helps synchronize the circadian rhythm, leading to improved sleep patterns.

Physical activity has also been shown to shorten the time it takes to fall asleep, reduce the number of overnight awakenings, and increase the overall duration of sleep.

Exercise also improves deeper, more peaceful sleep by lowering stress, anxiety, and tension, which are typical causes of sleep problems.

Furthermore, regular exercise might help reduce the symptoms of sleep problems like insomnia and sleep apnea. Exercise helps to promote relaxation, reduce daytime tiredness, and improve mood, all of which contribute to a better sleep experience.

In conclusion, including regular physical activity into your daily routine can result in greater sleep quality and overall health. Exercise is essential for comfortable and rejuvenating sleep because it promotes relaxation, reduces tension and anxiety, and supports the body's normal sleep-wake cycle.

Chapter 13: Tips for Implementing Physical Activity and Exercise:

1. Find Activities That You Enjoy:

Choose physical activities you enjoy and look forward to undertaking. Whether it's dancing, swimming, hiking, or sports, choosing activities that make you happy makes it simpler to stay motivated and committed.

Finding things   you enjoy is essential for sticking to a consistent and satisfying workout regimen. Exercise does not have to be a chore; it may be an opportunity to accomplish things that make you happy and satisfied.

There are numerous ways to stay active and fit, such as dancing, swimming, hiking, participating in sports, or practicing yoga.

You're more likely to stay motivated and committed to your fitness objectives if you choose activities you really enjoy.

When you are having fun, exercise becomes less of a chore and more of a fulfilling experience. It can be an opportunity to relax, de-stress, and refuel both physically and psychologically.

Experiment with several activities to see what resonates with you the most. Consider your interests, preferences, and personality qualities when choosing activities.

If you prefer being outside, consider hiking or riding. If you like to socialize, consider joining group fitness courses or recreational sports leagues. Alternatively, if you value isolation and reflection, yoga or swimming may be more appealing.

Remember that there is no one-size-fits-all method to exercise, so don't be afraid to experiment and try various things until you figure out what works best for you.

The idea is to put happiness first and choose activities that make you excited to be active. Incorporating activities   you enjoy into your routine will not only improve your physical health, but also your general well-being and quality of life.

2. Begin slowly and progress gradually

If you're new to exercise or haven't been active in a while, begin with low-impact activities and gradually increase the intensity and length. Listen to your body and avoid pushing yourself too hard, especially at the start.

When beginning a new fitness adventure, it is critical to start cautiously and improve steadily. It's tempting to get right into tough workouts or ambitious exercise routines, but doing too much too soon might lead to burnout, injury, or disappointment. Instead, a progressive approach allows your body to adapt and safely gain strength and endurance over time.

Set reasonable goals and build a foundation of consistent action. Begin with simple workouts that will challenge you without overwhelming you. For example, if you're new to running, begin with a mix of walking and jogging, gradually increasing your running intervals as your fitness improves.

Listen to your body and notice how you feel during and after exercise. It's acceptable to feel some muscle soreness or exhaustion, but if you feel severe pain or extreme discomfort, it's time to back off and reconsider your strategy.

As you progress, steadily increase the intensity, duration, and frequency of your workouts. This could include adding more weight to your strength training workouts, extending the duration of your cardio sessions, or adopting new and more difficult activities into your daily routine.

Remember that progress does not always follow a straight line, and there will be ups and downs. Be patient with yourself, and celebrate minor successes and milestones along the way.

By beginning slowly and gradually, you set yourself up for long-term success and sustainability in your fitness pursuits.

3. Set Realistic Goals:

Set achievable goals that align with your fitness level and lifestyle. Whether it's walking for 30 minutes a day, completing a 5k run, or mastering a new yoga pose, setting realistic goals helps keep you focused and motivated.

Setting attainable goals is critical for success in any undertaking. Realistic goals are ones that can be met within a reasonable time frame, taking into account one's resources, abilities, and limits. To properly track progress, goals should be explicit and quantitative.

To develop realistic goals, begin by evaluating your current condition and capabilities objectively. Understand your own talents and shortcomings, as well as the resources that are available to you. Consider any limitations or obstacles that may prevent you from achieving your objectives.

Then, state your goals clearly and specifically. Avoid creating unclear or unrealistic goals that are unlikely to be met. To make larger goals more achievable, break them down into smaller, doable tasks.

It is also critical to set timeframes for reaching your goals. This creates a sense of urgency and helps you stay focused on your efforts. Make sure you give yourself enough time to finish each work without becoming overwhelmed.

Review your goals on a regular basis and make any necessary adjustments. Circumstances may change, necessitating that you adjust your goals. Celebrate your victories along the journey, no matter how minor, and learn from any failures or problems you face.

Setting realistic goals and keeping committed to them can better prepare you to make meaningful progress and achieve success in your activities.

4. Add Variety:

To target different muscle groups and enhance overall fitness, incorporate a combination of cardiovascular, weight training, flexibility, and balancing exercises into your regimen. Variety not only keeps you from being bored, but it also lowers your chances of developing overuse problems.

Variety in your training regimen is critical for staying motivated, avoiding boredom, and obtaining peak fitness outcomes.

When you do the same exercises over and over again, your body adjusts to the actions, resulting in progress plateaus and declining returns.

You can keep your workouts new and fun by using a variety of exercises and activities that engage different muscle groups and prevent overuse issues.

There are numerous strategies to mix up your workout routine. Alternate between running, cycling, swimming, and high-intensity interval training to vary your cardio routines.

Include strength training movements that target specific muscle groups, such as squats, lunges, push-ups, and rows. To keep things exciting and fun, try out different fitness classes, sports, or outdoor activities.

Remember to incorporate activities that enhance flexibility, balance, and mobility, such as yoga, Pilates, or tai chi. These exercises not only supplement your strength and cardio routines, but they also help you avoid injuries and improve your overall physical performance.

By incorporating diversity into your training program, you will not only remain engaged and motivated, but you will also see better increases in strength, endurance, and general fitness.

Furthermore, you will have the opportunity to find new activities that you enjoy and anticipate, making fitness a sustainable and joyful part of your routine.

5. Make It Social

To make physical activity more fun and social, exercise with friends and family or participate in group fitness courses. Having a support system can help keep you accountable and motivated to stick to your workout plan.

Making exercise social can improve your motivation, enjoyment, and overall fitness experience. Working out with friends and family, or attending group fitness programs, helps you to share your journey to greater health and well-being while also building a sense of camaraderie and accountability.

Exercising with others allows for social engagement and connection, which can improve mood and decrease feelings of isolation or loneliness.

Whether it's playing a team sport, attending a group fitness class, or simply going for a stroll with a friend, exercising together fosters shared experiences and memories that improve connections and friendships.

Furthermore, exercising in a group can motivate and challenge you to push yourself harder than you would on your own. The excitement and encouragement from the other participants can drive you to attempt new things, set greater fitness goals, and stick to your fitness regimen.

Socializing while exercising can also make the experience more enjoyable and fun. Laughter, friendly competition, and shared triumphs foster a happy and supportive environment, making exercises feel more like a social gathering rather than a duty.

Whether you prefer the companionship of others or prefer to work out alone, including social aspects into your exercise regimen can increase your overall satisfaction, motivation, and adherence to regular physical activity.

So, grab a friend, sign up for a class, or organize a group workout to get the numerous benefits of making exercise sociable.

6. Prioritize Consistency

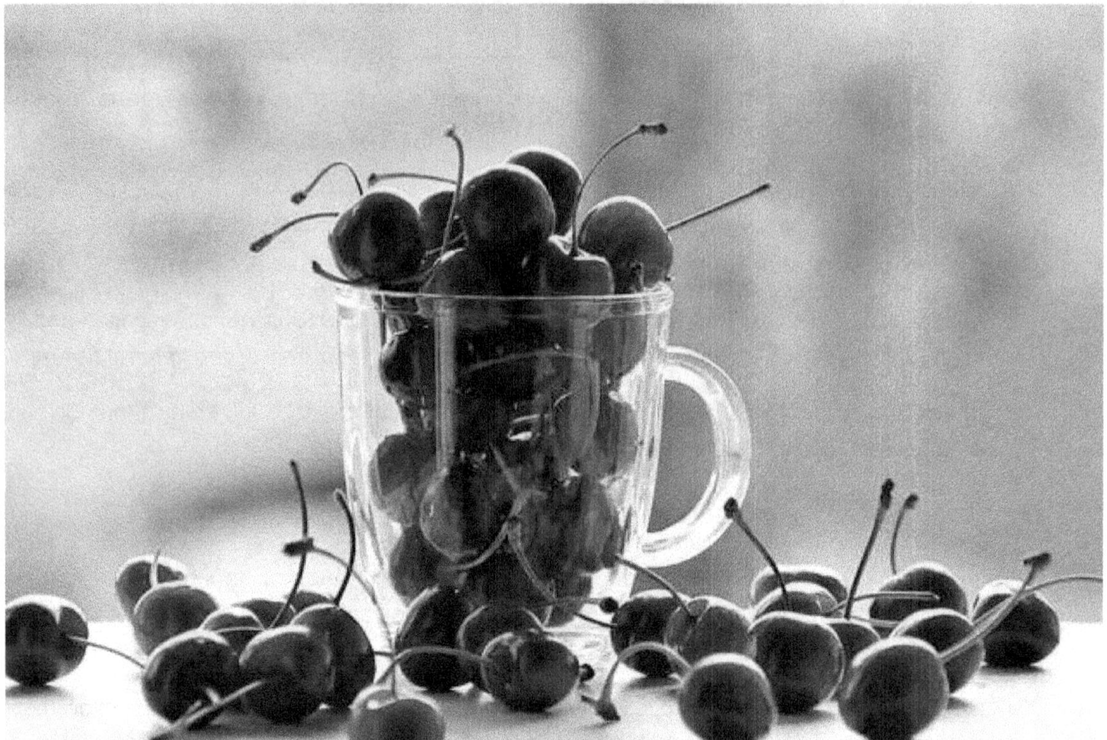

Instead of striving for perfection, focus on consistency. Even modest periods of physical activity throughout the day can build up and improve your overall health and fitness. Make exercise a mandatory element of your everyday regimen.

Consistency is the foundation of any good training plan, and it is critical to meeting your fitness goals. Prioritizing consistency is making exercise a non-negotiable component of your daily or weekly routine, regardless of external circumstances or impediments.

Consistency is essential because it allows you to gain momentum and advance toward your goals over time. Consistent exercise allows your body to adapt and enhance cardiovascular fitness, strength, endurance, flexibility, and general health.

Making exercise a regular habit builds discipline and commitment to your health and well-being. Even on days when you're not feeling motivated or energetic, adhering to your exercise regimen helps you retain momentum and avoid setbacks.

Furthermore, consistency produces outcomes. Over time, the cumulative effect of little, regular efforts results in considerable increases in fitness and general health. Consistently turning up for workouts, especially when they are difficult, fosters resilience, tenacity, and self-esteem.

Create a realistic fitness program that matches your lifestyle and commitments in order to prioritize regularity. Set precise goals, keep track of your progress, and hold yourself accountable. Find strategies to make exercise fun and sustainable, so you'll be more likely to stay with it in the long run.

Remember that consistency doesn't mean perfection. It's okay to have occasional setbacks or missed workouts; the key is to get back on track and stay consistent over the long term. By prioritizing consistency, you set yourself up for success in achieving your fitness goals and maintaining a healthy, active lifestyle.

7. Listen to Your Body:

Pay attention to how your body feels during and after exercise. If you experience pain or discomfort, modify your activities accordingly and seek guidance from a healthcare professional if needed.

Listening to your body is a fundamental principle of a healthy and sustainable approach to exercise and overall well-being.

Your body communicates its needs, limitations, and signals through sensations, feelings, and physical cues. By tuning in and paying attention to these messages, you can make informed decisions that support your health and fitness goals.

Listening to your body entails obeying its cues for hunger, fullness, exhaustion, and discomfort. It requires being aware of how different diets, workouts, and activities make you feel physically, psychologically, and emotionally.

For example, if you feel really exhausted or painful after a workout, it may be a warning that you should rest and recover rather than continuing with strenuous exercise.

Listening to your body also allows you to distinguish between typical discomfort caused by exertion and pain that may suggest injury or overtraining. It enables you to modify your exercise intensity, duration, and kind based on your body's signals in order to avoid injury and enhance recovery.

Finally, listening to your body promotes a deeper connection and knowledge of your physical and emotional needs, resulting in increased self-awareness, balance, and general well-being.

By acknowledging and respecting your body's messages, you may create a positive and long-term connection with exercise and nutrition, boosting overall health and vitality.

To summarize, physical activity and exercise are necessary components of a healthy lifestyle. By implementing regular physical activity into your daily routine and prioritizing it, you can enjoy numerous physical and mental health benefits. Remember that every step you take helps you become a better, happier person.

Chapter 14: Mind set and Behavior Changes

Achieving and maintaining your target weight entails more than just dietary and exercise adjustments; it also necessitates a transformation in mentality and behavior. Consider the following ways to encourage long-term habit change:

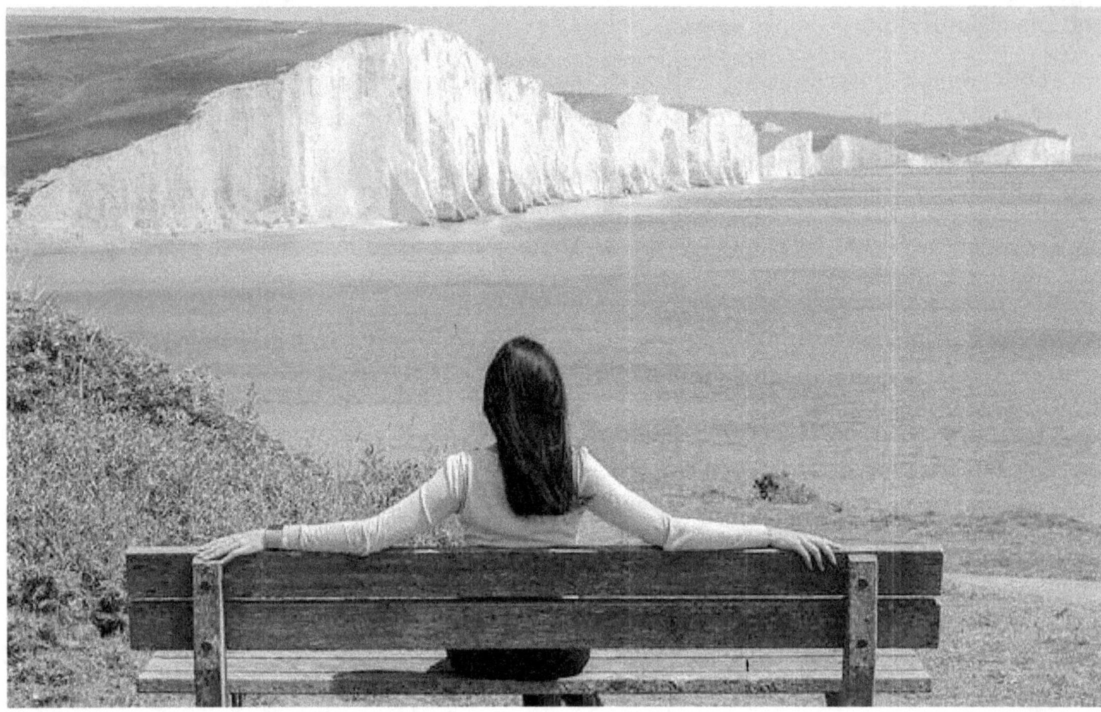

Unlocking Potential: The Power of Change in Mind set and Behavior

Mind set and behavior change are the driving forces that determine our experiences and outcomes on the path to personal growth and self-improvement.

From reaching job goals to leading a healthy lifestyle, how we perceive challenges and approach change has a huge impact on our ability to achieve our objectives.

In this in-depth examination, we will delve into the tremendous impact of thought and behavior transformation, comprehending their dynamics and revealing ways for capitalizing on their transforming potential.

Understanding Mind sets:

Carol Dweck invented the term "mind set" to describe our ideas and attitudes toward ourselves, our skills, and the world around us. According to Dweck's research, there are two major mind sets: fixed and growth.

1. The Fixed Mind set

People who have a fixed mind set feel that their abilities, intelligence, and capabilities are inherent and immutable. They see problems as a threat to their self-esteem and shun them in order to maintain their sense of competence.

Failure is viewed as a reflection of their fundamental limits, resulting in sentiments of powerlessness and resignation.

2. The Growth Mind set:

Those with a growth mentality, on the other hand, see setbacks as opportunities for personal and professional development. They believe that abilities can be acquired via hard work, practice, and perseverance.

Individuals with a   growth mentality view losses as stepping stones to achievement, demonstrating resilience, optimism, and a desire to take on new tasks.

The effect of mind set on behavior change:

Our mind set has a significant impact on our behavior and behaviors, influencing how we respond to challenges and failures. Consider two people going on a weight loss journey.

Fixed Mind set:

A person with a fixed mind set may approach weight reduction with a rigid set of beliefs, perceiving setbacks like a missed workout or an excessive meal as proof of their unwillingness to change. As a result, they may give up quickly, succumbing to feelings of frustration and failure.

Growth Mind set:

On the other hand, someone with a development mentality tackles weight loss with an open mind, seeing setbacks as opportunities for reflection and improvement.

They understand that growth is not linear and are open to changing their approach depending on feedback and experience. As a result, they endure through obstacles and eventually succeed.

Chapter 15: Promoting a Growth Mind set:

While attitude may appear to be fixed, it can be fostered and nurtured with purposeful effort and practice. Here are several approaches to cultivating a growth mind set:

1. Be open to challenges:

Instead of avoiding problems, view them as chances for growth and self-improvement. Maintain a "can-do" attitude and face challenges with curiosity and resilience.

2. See Effort as the Path to Mastery:

Recognize that perseverance is the key to mastery and success. Accept the process of learning and development, putting effort and dedication ahead of intrinsic talent.

3. Get Feedback:

Consider every feedback, good or negative, to be vital information for personal development. Use constructive criticism to help you improve and refine your skills.

4. Recognize and celebrate growth and progress.

Recognize and appreciate your development and accomplishments, no matter how minor. Cultivate a grateful and optimistic mind set, concentrating on the journey of self-discovery and growth.

Chapter 16: Behavior Change: The Path to Transformation

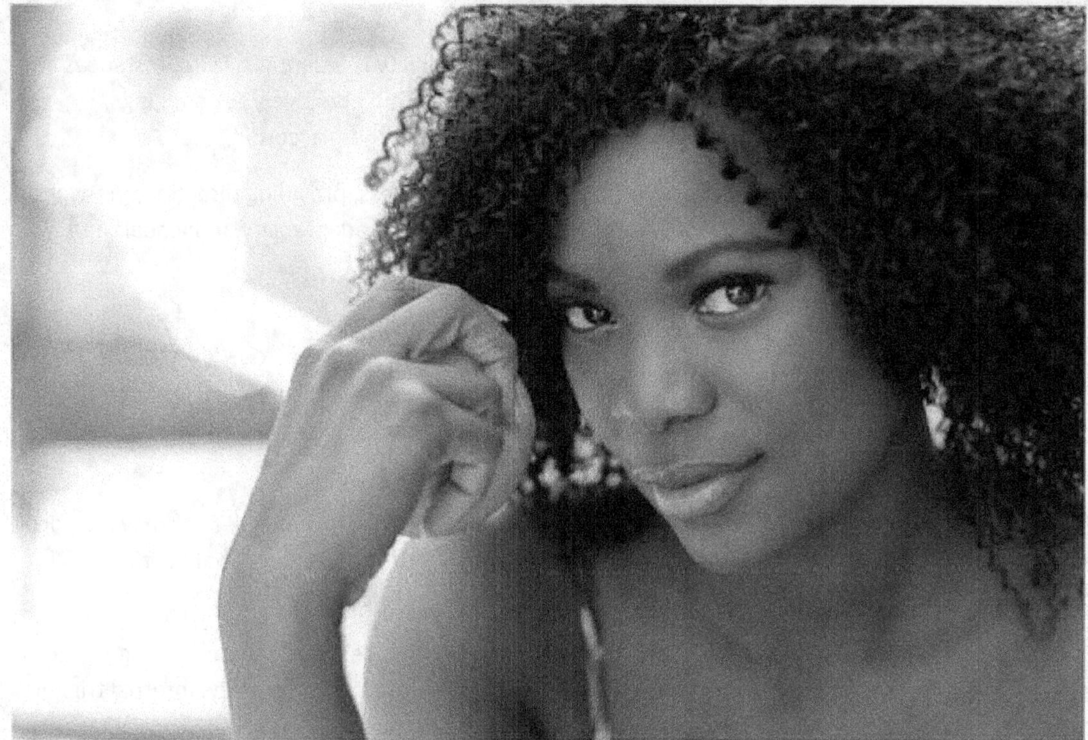

Behavior modification is the process of forming new habits or adjusting old ones in order to attain a certain goal. Whether it's stopping smoking, eating healthier, or improving time management skills, behavior change necessitates a thoughtful and methodical approach.

1. Set Clear and Achievable Goals:

Set explicit, quantifiable goals that are both realistic and achievable. Break down huge goals into smaller, more doable tasks to keep momentum and track progress.

Setting specific, attainable goals is an essential strategy for success in any undertaking. Clear goals provide direction, focus, and motivation, driving individuals or teams to the intended outcomes. These goals act as milestones along the way, allowing us to track our progress and celebrate our accomplishments.

To set precise goals, they must be defined specifically. Vague aims can cause confusion and a lack of clarity. Each goal should be well-defined, indicating exactly what has to be completed, who will do it, and when. This clarity helps to eliminate uncertainty and ensures that everyone involved knows the goal.

Furthermore, goals must be achievable. While it is necessary to aim high, adopting unreasonable goals can be discouraging and unproductive.

Assessing resources, capabilities, and schedules is critical for determining the feasibility of a task. Break down huge goals into smaller, more achievable activities to make progress more visible and realistic.

Furthermore, goals should be consistent with overall objectives, whether personal, professional, or organizational. This alignment ensures that actions contribute significantly to larger goals, promoting coherence and synergy.

Regular assessment and revision of goals is also required. Flexibility is essential as circumstances and priorities alter. Individuals and teams can stay on track and respond effectively to changing circumstances by reassessing goals on a regular basis and revising them accordingly.

In essence, setting clear, achievable goals is a cornerstone of success, providing direction, motivation, and a roadmap for progress. With clarity, feasibility, alignment, and adaptability, individuals and teams can navigate challenges and realize their aspirations.

2. Identify Triggers and Barriers:

Understand the triggers and obstacles that influence your behavior. Anticipate challenges and develop strategies to overcome them, whether it's avoiding temptation, seeking social support, or managing stress.

Triggers can vary greatly depending on the context and individual circumstances. They may include external factors such as environmental cues, social situations, or specific events that prompt a particular reaction.

For example, seeing a tempting dessert might trigger cravings for sweets in someone trying to stick to a healthy diet, or receiving a critical email might trigger feelings of stress or anxiety. Internal triggers, such as emotions, thoughts, or physical sensations, can also play a significant role.

For instance, feeling lonely might trigger a desire for social interaction, or experiencing fatigue might trigger procrastination.

Barriers, on the other hand, are barriers that impede progress or prohibit people from achieving their objectives. These impediments may be internal or external.

Internal hurdles can include self-doubt, a lack of enthusiasm, or a fear of failure, whereas external barriers can be money limits, time constraints, or a lack of access to resources. For example, a single parent attempting to take evening classes to enhance their degree may encounter a shortage of childcare options, while a language barrier may impede communication in a multicultural workplace.

Identifying triggers and barriers is critical for creating effective strategies for managing behavior and overcoming obstacles. Individuals can implement targeted interventions to address the factors that prompt certain behaviors or impede progress,

Allowing them to work more effectively toward their goals. This could entail implementing coping mechanisms to deal with triggers or devising solutions to overcome specific barriers through problem-solving and resourcefulness.

3. Create a Supportive Environment

Surround yourself with people, resources, and environments that will support and reinforce your desired behaviors. Seek out social support, accountability partners, and role models who will inspire and motivate you.

Creating a supportive environment entails setting up conditions and resources that promote individual or group growth, well-being, and success. This environment should be supportive, inclusive, and encouraging of personal and group development.

Promoting open communication and collaboration is an important part of developing a supportive atmosphere. Encouragement of open communication and attentive listening contributes to individual trust and understanding.

Regular team meetings, one-on-one check-ins, and the creation of channels for sharing ideas and comments can all help to achieve this.

Another critical component is making available tools and opportunities for skill development and learning. This could include providing training programs, workshops, or access to educational materials that enable people to improve their knowledge and capacities.

Furthermore, mentoring or coaching can offer direction and support as individuals strive towards their goals.

Creating a physically and emotionally safe setting is also critical. This includes making sure the physical space is comfortable and accessible, as well as instilling a culture of respect and understanding.

It is critical to respond quickly and effectively to any incidences of discrimination or harassment in order to preserve a supportive environment.

Furthermore, recognizing and celebrating achievements and milestones helps to foster a pleasant and motivated workplace. Recognizing individuals' efforts and accomplishments maintains a sense of worth and promotes continuous growth and participation.

Overall, developing a supportive environment necessitates a comprehensive approach that addresses individuals' physical, emotional, and developmental needs while also instilling a sense of belonging, empowerment, and mutual support.

4. Develop Self-Compassion:

Be kind with yourself throughout the process of changing your behaviors. Accept that setbacks are an unavoidable part of the road and treat yourself with compassion and respect. Instead than being markers of failure, view setbacks as chances for learning and progress.

Self-compassion is the practice of treating oneself with kindness, understanding, and acceptance, particularly during times of adversity or pain. It necessitates accepting one's own humanity and flaws without condemnation or self-criticism.

One aspect of self-compassion is cultivating a mindset of self-kindness. This involves speaking to oneself in a gentle and supportive manner, much like one would comfort a friend facing a challenge.

Instead of berating oneself for mistakes or shortcomings, self-kindness encourages offering words of encouragement and reassurance.

Another important component is recognizing common humanity. Understanding that everyone experiences setbacks, failures, and struggles at some point in their lives helps put one's own experiences into perspective.

This realization fosters a sense of connection with others and reduces feelings of isolation or inadequacy.

Furthermore, mindfulness plays a key role in practicing self-compassion. Being present in the moment and observing one's thoughts and emotions without judgment allows for greater self-awareness and emotional regulation.

Mindfulness practices such as meditation or deep breathing can help cultivate a sense of calm and perspective.

Overall, practicing self-compassion involves treating oneself with the same kindness, understanding, and empathy that one would extend to others. By embracing self-compassion, individuals can cultivate resilience, self-esteem, and overall well-being, leading to a more fulfilling and balanced life.

5. Be Consistent and Persistent

Behavior modification relies heavily on consistency. Even when confronted with obstacles or disappointments, remain committed to your goals and focus your efforts. Maintain your long-term vision and persist in your pursuit of change.

Maintaining consistency and persistence is essential for attaining long-term objectives and overcoming difficulties. Consistency is defined as maintaining a consistent effort or habit across time, whereas perseverance is defined as continuing to pursue a goal in the face of setbacks or problems.

Consistency is important because it allows for the slow accumulation of development and momentum. Individuals can develop habits, abilities, and momentum that carry them toward their goals by continuously showing up and putting in the effort.

Consistency, whether it's practicing a new skill on a daily basis, sticking to a workout program, or pursuing a professional goal, helps to cement progress and bring you closer to achievement.

Persistence is equally crucial since it allows people to overcome setbacks and challenges. It entails tenacity in the face of adversity, the ability to learn from failures, and the determination to persevere despite setbacks.

When confronted with hurdles or disappointments, persistence motivates people to adapt, problem solve, and continue until they achieve their goal.

Consistency and persistence work together to create a tremendous force that propels progress and success. Consistently showing up and putting in effort,

combined with the desire to persevere in the face of adversity, increases the likelihood of attaining goals and realizing aspirations. Individuals can achieve their goals by staying devoted to them and remaining resilient in the face of hardship.

Chapter 17: Combining Mind set and Behavior Change:

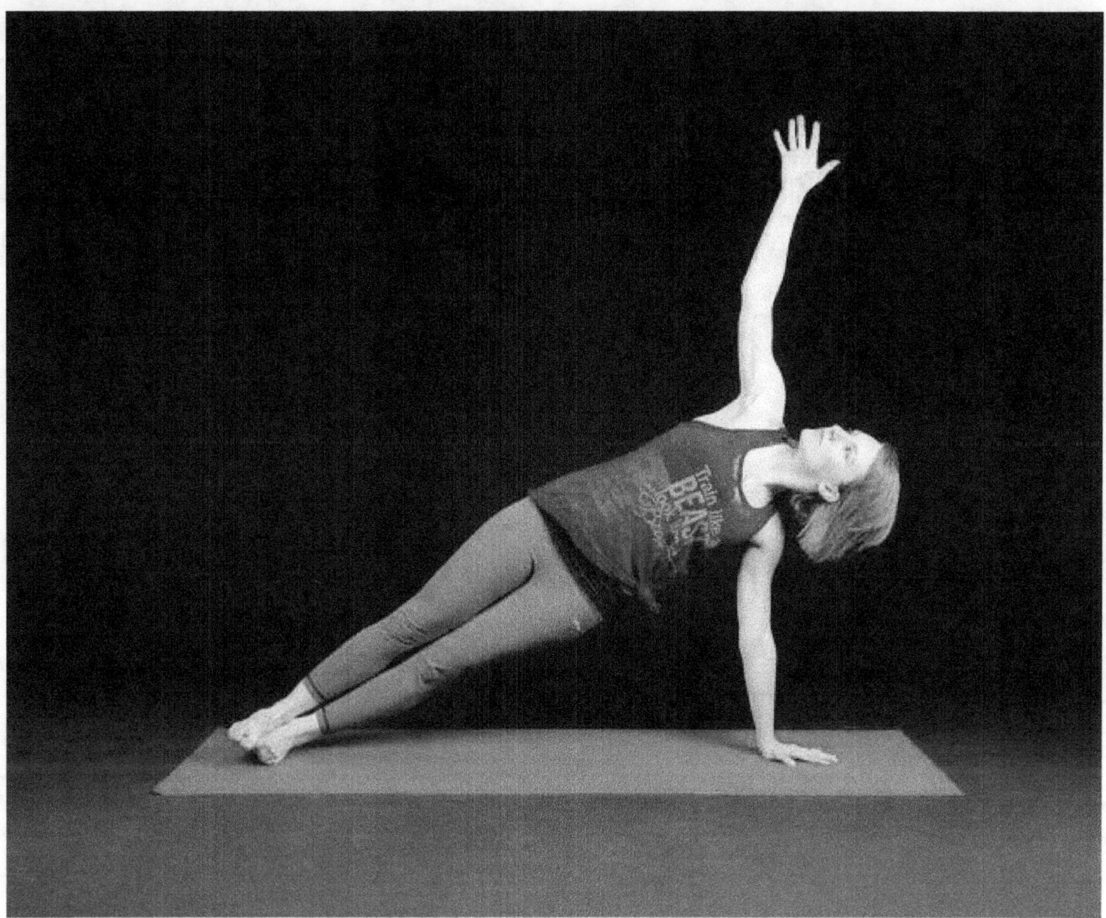

It is impossible to deny that thought and behavior transformation work together. A growth mind set serves as the foundation for launching and maintaining behavior change attempts, while behavior change reinforces and develops the growth mentality. Consider the following scenario:

Integrating mind set and behavior change entails matching one's thoughts, beliefs, and attitudes with deliberate actions and behaviors in order to accomplish desired results.

This approach necessitates a thorough grasp of how attitude effects behavior and vice versa, as well as deliberate tactics for cultivating a mind set conducive to positive transformation.

To begin, individuals must identify and address any limiting beliefs or negative thought patterns that may be impeding behavior change. This entails fostering a growth mentality, which sees problems as chances for advancement and believes in one's potential to learn and better over time.

Individuals who adopt a growth mind set are more likely to approach behavior change with optimism, resilience, and a readiness to try new approaches.

Secondly, integrating mind set and behavior change involves setting clear, achievable goals and developing action plans to support them. By breaking down larger goals into smaller, manageable steps, individuals can create a roadmap for behavior change and track their progress over time.

This process encourages accountability and provides a sense of direction, making it easier to stay motivated and focused on long-term success.

Additionally, practicing mindfulness and self-awareness can facilitate integration between mind set and behavior change.

By cultivating present-moment awareness and observing thoughts and emotions without judgment, individuals can gain insight into the underlying drivers of their behavior and make conscious choices aligned with their desired outcomes.

Overall, integrating mind set and behavior change requires a holistic approach that addresses both cognitive and behavioral aspects. By cultivating a growth mind set, setting clear goals, and practicing mindfulness, individuals can empower themselves to make lasting changes and achieve their full potential.

Mind set:

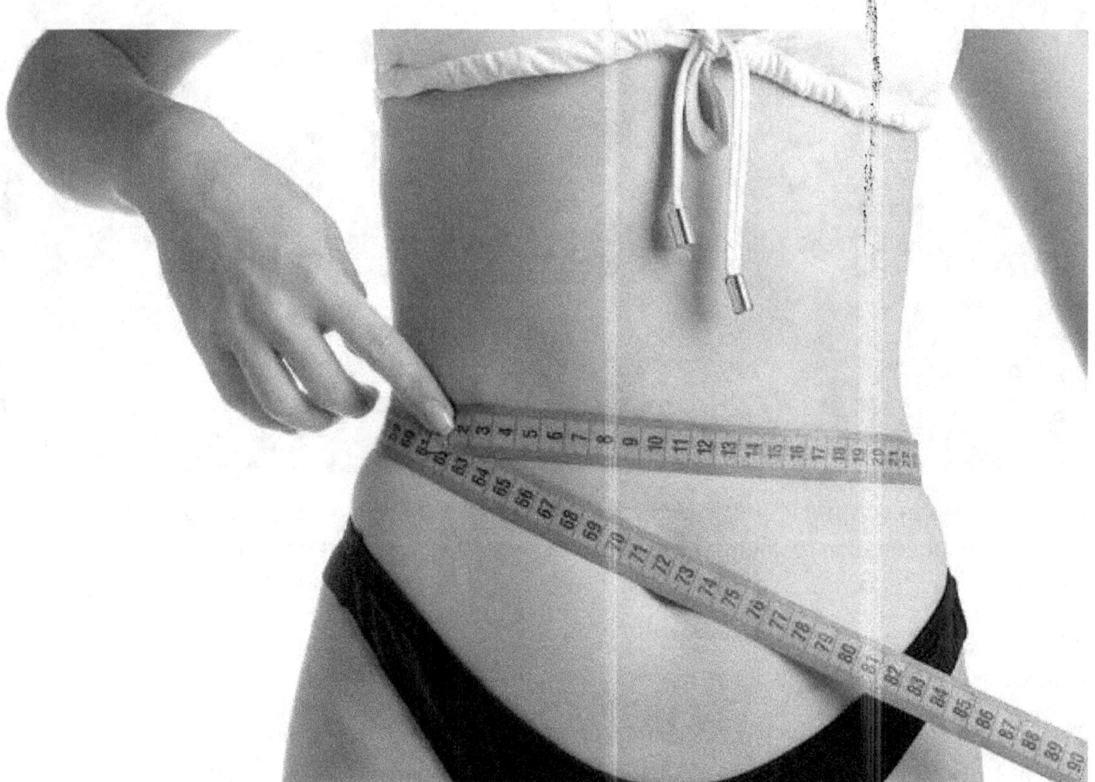

A growth mind set prepares people to accept the process of behavior change, seeing problems as chances for growth and learning. It fosters resilience, optimism, and confidence in one's potential to change.

Mind set is the established collection of attitudes, ideas, and assumptions that influence how people view themselves, others, and the world around them. It determines how people face obstacles, deal with adversity, and achieve their goals.

A growth mentality accepts that abilities and intelligence may be acquired by hard work and perseverance, whereas a fixed mind set believes that traits are innate and unchanging.

Cultivating a growth mind set promotes resilience, perseverance, and a readiness to learn, allowing people to adapt, grow, and prosper in the face of challenges and disappointments.

Behavioral Change:

Active participation in behavior change attempts fosters a growth mind set by offering concrete evidence of progress and accomplishment. Small victories and accomplishments confirm the assumption that effort leads to improvement, maintaining the cycle of growth and self-efficacy.

Behavior modification is the process of changing actions, habits, or patterns of behavior in order to accomplish desired results or increase overall well-being. It entails intentionally adopting new behaviors or removing current ones with deliberate effort and desire.

Setting precise goals, developing practical plans, and executing techniques to overcome barriers or obstacles are all common requirements for successful behavior change.

Whether it's adopting healthier lifestyle habits, increasing time management skills, or breaking bad behaviors, behavior change necessitates self-awareness, dedication, and determination.

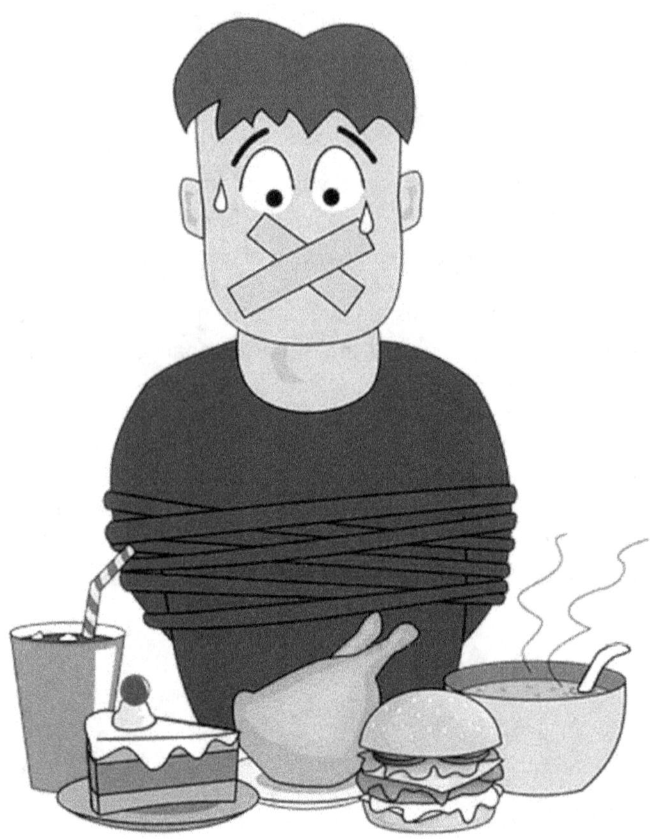

Conclusion:

To summarize, obtaining your target weight is a journey that involves dedication, perseverance, and a comprehensive strategy.

It's not just about sticking to a tight diet or putting in long hours at the gym; it's about implementing long-term lifestyle adjustments that promote overall health and wellness.

This process entails forming healthier eating habits, remaining physically active, effectively managing stress, and emphasizing self-care.

Furthermore, achieving your ideal weight is more than just a number on the scale; it is also about how you feel physically, psychologically, and emotionally.

It's all about developing a positive connection with food, accepting your body's normal swings, and practicing self-compassion along the way.

Importantly, requesting help from friends, family, or healthcare experts can provide vital encouragement and guidance along the way. Remember that setbacks are unavoidable, and it's critical to approach them with resilience and growth mentality.

Finally, the journey to your optimum weight is unique to you, and it is critical to focus on progress rather than perfection. Celebrate your successes, no matter how modest, and remain devoted to your long-term health and pleasure.

You may achieve your goals and live a full life in a body that feels strong, energized, and balanced if you practice patience, persistence, and a good attitude.

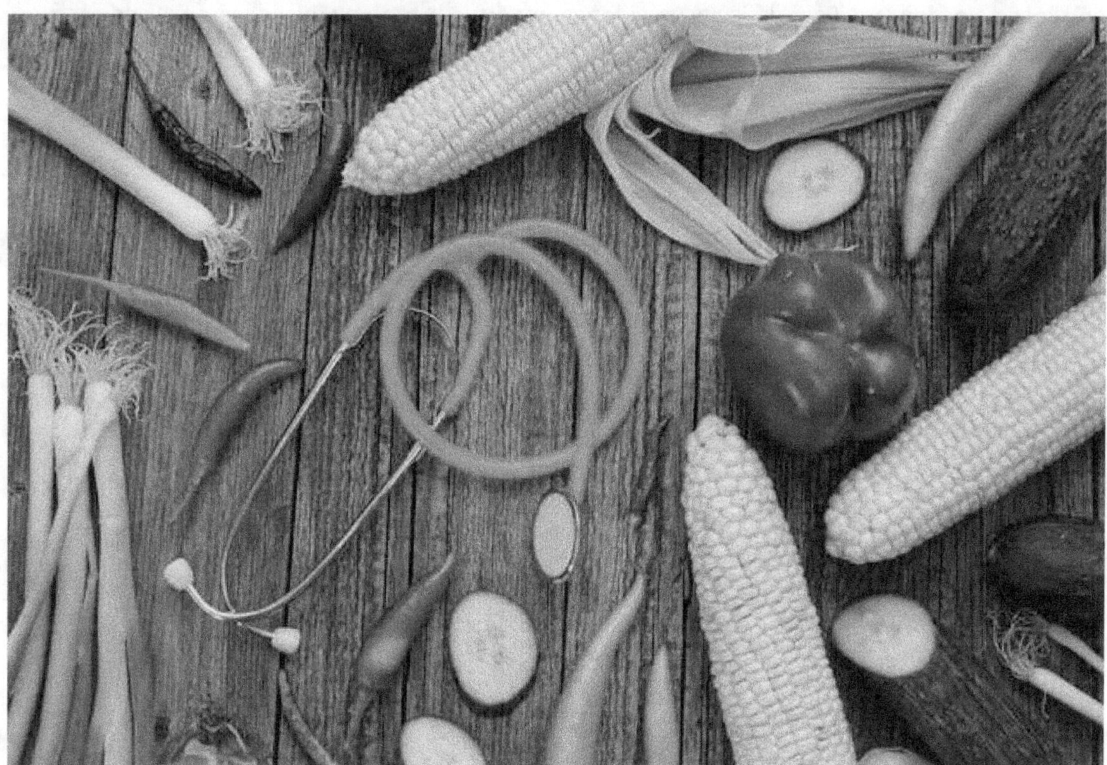

AUTHOR'S NOTE

Dear Readers

THERE IS LOT TO EXPERIENCE IN LIFETIME – START EXPLORE!!

As you embark on your path to success, keep in mind that you have the ability to attain your goals and desires. You will have challenges and setbacks along the way, but it is critical that you remain resilient and keep going forward. Each difficulty provides an opportunity for growth and learning, and each step puts you closer to your objectives.

Be confident in yourself and your ability. You are capable of great things, and your distinct abilities and characteristics have the ability to positively impact the world around you. Accept your full potential and dare to dream large.

Find inspiration in the stories of people who overcame adversity and succeeded despite the odds. Their stories serve as reminders that with determination, perseverance, and hard work, anything is possible.

Surround yourself with happiness and encouragement. Seek for mentors, friends, and colleagues who can encourage and motivate you on your journey. Their advice, wisdom, and support can give you the inspiration you need to keep going, even when things get rough.

Remember to acknowledge your progress and accomplishments along the way, no matter how minor they may appear. Each achievement is a credit to your hard work and commitment.

Above all, trust in the journey and have faith in yourself. Believe that you are deserving of success and that your efforts will be rewarded in due time. Keep striving, keep believing, and never lose sight of the vision you have for your life.

You are capable, you are resilient, and you are destined for greatness. Let your journey be guided by courage, optimism, and a relentless pursuit of your dreams. The world is waiting for you to shine your light brightly and make your mark. Keep going, keep growing, and never lose sight of the incredible potential that lies within you.

(104)

With warmest wishes for your success.

[Ms. Anusha]